THE ADMINISTRATION
OF A PUBLIC HEALTH AGENCY

THE ADMINISTRATION OF A PUBLIC HEALTH AGENCY

*A Case Study
of the New York City
Department of Health*

Pascal James Imperato, M.D.

*State University of New York
Downstate Medical Center,
New York*

HUMAN SCIENCES PRESS, INC.
72 FIFTH AVENUE,
NEW YORK, N.Y. 10011

Copyright © 1983 by Human Sciences Press, Inc.
72 Fifth Avenue, New York, New York 10011

Printed in the United States of America
23456789 987654321

Library of Congress Cataloging in Publication Data

Imperato, Pascal James.
    The administration of a public health agency.

    Bibliography: p.
    Includes index.
    1. New York (City).   Dept. of Health—History.
2 Public health administration—New York (City)—History.
I. Title
RA121.I46   1983   352.94'41'097471   83–31
ISBN 0-89885-122-X

Dedicated
with Permission
to
His Majesty
King Humbert II of Italy
with Affection
and Grateful Appreciation

Table of Contents

PREFACE

The principal focus of this book is on the New York City Department of Health during the late 1960s and the 1970s. This fifteen-year period witnessed enormous social, political, and economic changes not only in New York City, but throughout the United States. The civil rights movement, the anti-Viet Nam war protest movement, and agitation on the part of youth for sweeping social, political, and economic changes produced great upheavals in time-honored American institutions, attitudes, and values. These were not without effect on the Department of Health and its missions. By the mid-1970s the driving forces of this major upheaval had spent themselves. However, they left a legacy of new programs, changed values and attitudes, and altered governmental structures that had been created to meet their demands.

Although federal, state, and local initiatives for dealing with a host of urban problems had slowed by the early 1970s, it was not until 1975 that they came to an almost abrupt halt in New York City because of the fiscal crisis. The fiscal crisis fell upon a city whose independent home rule was already being eroded by forces tending to centralize power and authority at the state level. All of these events had a dramatic effect on both the structure and functions of the Department of Health and on those who led it during these years.

The Health Services Administration was a superagency created in 1966 in the hope of more effectively dealing with the needs and wants of New Yorkers, particularly the urban poor. For the first time in its history, the Department of Health found itself part of a larger formal city health structure with its commissioner reporting not to the mayor, but to a health administrator. By 1973 this new experiment had run its course and had fallen out of favor as a reasonable approach. But times had also changed nationally, moving from the era of ever-expanding horizons to one of recognized limits. Thus, the 1970s initially witnessed structural changes again, with the disman-

9

tling of the Health Services Administration and the restoration of the Department of Health to its former position. But, obviously, for a number of reasons, that position was not the same as before.

The diffusion of public health functions into a host of federal, state, and local agencies other than public health departments took place at an accelerated pace during the 1970s. New York City was no exception. Around the country, public health departments became increasingly residuary in nature, consisting of potpourri functions unwanted by other agencies. And these functions were often not on the cutting edge of public health. Separate agencies were created for environmental problems, occupational health, substance abuse, mental health, and even health planning. This national trend in governance change of public health functions was strongly resisted by public health officials in New York City with considerable success. But it remained an ongoing struggle, waged simultaneously against attempts to centralize public health functions at the state level. If this were not enough, city health commissioners then had to deal with the worst fiscal crisis in New York City's history and had to preserve the department's structural and functional integrity while under the cloud of looming bankruptcy.

Having ceded financial control to the state in everything but name, the city lost a great degree of its autonomy at a point in history when the forces of state centralization were growing in strength. It was at this time that the city and state were forced to deal with the politically hazardous issue of the municipal hospitals grouped under the Health and Hospitals Corporation. Running enormous deficits not only because of managerial problems but, more important, because of larger social and economic problems, these hospitals presented problems that defied easy solutions. Having amassed the necessary power and authority over hospitals during better days, the state was not unwilling to exercise them because of the predictable political hazards. What then ensued was an elaborate scheme to create a health czar, several steps removed from the state's governor, to deal with these hospital problems. State officials here saw an opportunity to make a final sweeping assault on the Department of Health. This attempt led to a protracted struggle in which the Department of Health preserved its independence.

Virtually every decade in the Department of Health's history has had its share of major problems, crises, and administrative challenges. What sets the late 1960s and 1970s apart from what took place before is the fact that the department also had to meet challenges that threatened its structural and functional integrity. In a sense, this book is an account of how the department and its professionals met these unusual challenges. In putting this account together, I have drawn upon three principal types of sources. These include a wealth of published materials, the impressions of a number of public health professionals who worked in the department during the fifteen-year period under study, and my own observations, made over the six-year period 1972 to 1978, when I served in the department.

I want to express my thanks to the many people who assisted me in the preparation of this book. I am especially grateful to Dr. Lowell E. Bellin, Dr. Mary C. McLaughlin, and Dr. Ernest L. Stebbins, all former health commissioners, who provided me with much useful information and many valuable insights. I am also grateful to Dr. Arthur Bushel who, having served as Acting Commissioner of Health in 1966, was familiar with the background to the creation of the Health Services Administration. I owe a very special debt of gratitude to Mr. Louis Neugeborn, former Deputy Commissioner for Administrative Services, who, having served in the department for over forty years, was a valuable source of information about its structure and functions and its long and complicated history from the 1940s through the end of the 1970s. I want to thank Mr. Harry Hollander and Mr. Irving Witlin, both of whom served as the department's General Counsel, and who gave me many useful insights based on their collective decades of first-hand experience. I also want to acknowledge the helpful assistance of Miss Helen Stone, former Director of Public Information for the department, Dr. Florence Kavaler, former Assistant Commissioner of Health, and Dr. Shirley Mayer, former First Deputy Commissioner of Health.

Dr. Howard Rusk, Director of the Institute of Rehabilitation Medicine, New York University Medical Center, has been a steadfast supporter, for which I am grateful. I also want to thank him for his counsel and advice during my years of service in the Department of Health.

The staff of the Downstate Medical Center Library and Mr. Sol Becker and the staff of the Haven Emerson Library at the Department of Health provided much valuable help. I also wish to thank the *Bulletin of the New York Academy of Medicine* for permission to use previously published material in preparing Chapter 5.

And to my wife Eleanor and my children Alison and Gavin I owe special thanks for their patience during the seemingly long period this book was in preparation. I am also grateful to my wife for having read and corrected numerous drafts of the manuscript.

Finally, I would like to thank Ms. Phyllis Alexander, Mrs. Mary Horn, Mrs. Constance Jones, Mrs. Eunice McKinney, and Mrs. Maureen Roaldsen for their careful preparation of the typescript.

Pascal James Imperato, M.D.

Chapter 1

AN OVERVIEW OF NEW YORK CITY

New York City has long been the largest city in the United States and one of the most complex in the world. It has been characterized as sixty cities in one because of its ethnic diversity, range of commercial and manufacturing activities, and spectrum of cultural institutions and events.[1] Its population is greater than those of the majority of states, and it has representation from almost every country in the world. Because of this ethnic diversity, the city has been called "the melting pot" by some.[2] Sophistication, wealth, and upwardly mobile opportunities were long-perceived attributes of the city. These perceptions had their roots in a reality characterized by steady economic expansion, better than average per capita income, and the growth of cultural and intellectual institutions.

But this reality began to change, slowly at first after World War II and then rapidly in the 1960s and on through the 1970s. Perception and understanding of this change were slow, even after the city had undergone obviously significant changes. It was not until the public unfolding of the city's fiscal crisis in 1975 that many realized New York City was no longer the place they thought it to be. What occurred in New York City was a complex process of decline, with diverse roots but characterized by a changing population, the erosion of the city's commercial and manufacturing infrastructure, a shrinkage in its intellectual and cultural life, and a deterioration of its very physical substance. Shocking and sobering though this may sound, it nonetheless took place and has not yet been reversed.[3] It is well to remember that municipal decline is not a uniquely New York City

13

phenomenon, but one which has taken place in a number of America's older northern cities, including Baltimore, Cleveland, Detroit and St. Louis.

The impact of this decline on public health and on public health services was enormous.[4] Thus an understanding of the city's recent history is necessary to a discussion of the administration of its public health agency. This history does not merely chronicle the process of decline, but also the responses of a local government to a broad spectrum of newer social, economic and health problems of a national nature.

NEW YORK AND ITS POPULATION

In 1970, New York City had a population of 7.8 million living in five boroughs covering three hundred square miles. By 1980, the population had dropped to 7.0 million, representing a loss of almost a million people. This contrasted with a 1.4 percent increase in the city's population between 1960 and 1970.[5] Although a major shift in the city's population had been underway in the 1950's, it was really in the 1960's that a middle class exodus became substantial. This exodus continued through the 1970's. In essence, these two decades witnessed the steady departure of black and white middle class populations and their replacement by poor black and hispanic groups, both from other areas of the United States and from other countries. Between 1960 and 1970, the black population of the Bronx rose 118 percent, that of Brooklyn 76 percent, Queens 77 percent and Richmond 63 percent. Manhattan's black population declined by 4 percent during this period. The hispanic population of the four outer boroughs similarly rose during the 1960's. By 1970 it had risen 70 percent in the Bronx, 51 percent in Brooklyn, 90 percent in Queens and 93 percent in Richmond. It fell by 18 percent in Manhattan.[6]

The 1980 census showed a continuation of these trends, but with an overall decline in the city's total population to 7,071,030, representing a decline of eleven percent. This decline was not unique in the state as a number of upstate counties containing large urban centers also lost population.

The city's black population rose slightly from 1,668,115 in 1970 to 1,784,124 in 1980, representing respectively 21% and 24.4% of the total. Although the white population of the city is listed as 4,293,695 for 1980 (61%) compared to 6,048,841 (77%) for 1970, this figure is misleading as many hispanics listed themselves as white and some under the category "other" of which 749,882 were recorded in 1980. It is estimated that half of this latter group is composed of hispanics and that the remaining 1,405,957 hispanics are listed as white. Given these facts the white population, exclusive of hispanics was about 3,257,738 in 1980, or 46.5% of the total. The black population was 1,784,124 or 24.4% and the hispanic, 1,405,957 or 20.1%. Other groups, including Asian and American Indians amounted to 623,211 or 8.9%. For the first time in the city's history non-white minorities formed the majority population.[7]

Additionally, it is estimated that anywhere from a half million to a million and a half illegal aliens lived in New York City at any given time during the 1970's.[8] Most were immigrants from Central and South America and the Caribbean.

EMPLOYMENT TRENDS

In 1970, there were approximately 3.75 million people employed in the city.[9] By 1977 that figure had dropped to 3.16 million, representing a loss of almost 600,000 jobs.[10] Betwen 1960 and 1970, the city lost 181,000 manufacturing jobs, compensated for by a gain of the same magnitude in service jobs. The annual loss of manufacturing jobs post-1970 has been in the order of 44,000.[11] During the five year period, 1970-1974, some 83,000 sales jobs and 36,500 jobs in finance, insurance and real estate were lost.[12] During the same time there was a gain of 33,500 jobs in government and 10,500 jobs in the service sector.[13] Morris has observed that the city's unemployment rate during the early 1970's rose by 83.6 percent, representing the highest in the country. In addition, the service and government jobs gained scarcely offset the jobs lost. Worse still, as far as the city's tax revenues were concerned, the jobs gained produced only half the amount of income taxes as an equal number of those lost. Morris points out that if a government job is assigned a tax yield value of 1, a services sector job would have a value of 1.44, a manufacturing job 1.60, a wholesale or retail trades job, 2.26 and a job in finance, insurance or real estate, a value of 2.66. Thus, it would take 2.66 government jobs to generate the tax revenues produced by one job in finance, insurance or real estate.[14]

The reasons for the city's continuous loss of jobs are many. Few would argue that the high corporate and personal income taxes levied by both New York City and New York State play a small role in causing the flight of businesses from the city. It is significant that a large number of businesses and corporate headquarters moved to nearby Connecticut where there is no state income tax and to New Jersey where there was also none until the late 1970's. But there were also a number of other reasons for the flight of commerce and industry. Auletta in documenting the reasons for the departure of Union Carbide from the city cites crime, high living costs, discomfort with the city's changing ethnic mix, the decline of basic city services, vandalism and dirt on the streets.[15] This is a rather sweeping indictment against the city, but it does not fully explain why businesses have left. The fact that commerce and industry can be profitably conducted in decentralized locations thanks to computers and modern highways coupled to the suburbanization of America and the individual's reliance on automobiles have had no small impact on the decline of all older northern cities. There has also been a massive shift of people and businesses out of the Northeast to the southern and western "sun-belt" areas. This redistribution has had especially negative economic effects on the Northeast. In the mid-1970's, the New York State Economic Development Board reported that the real income of the average citizen of the state was 1 percent below the national mean. And by the late 1970's, employment in the Northeast was increasing by only 2.1 percent, three times slower than in any other region of the country.[16]

HOUSING

Two major trends in housing characterized the 1970's. The most visible to outsiders and visitors was the surge of office, hotel and apartment building in Manhattan, particularly after 1975. Yet, it is far less significant than the massive abandonment of buildings by landlords and widespread arson of housing stock in the Bronx, Queens and Brooklyn. The Manhattan building boom is in a sense an artificiality, reflecting not the inherent fiscal health of the city, but rather a response to the city's tax abatement policies, a growing tourist industry and the investment of ex-patriated petro-dollars and other wealth from abroad. No one will argue that new construction in Manhattan is better than none. But it is the result of stimuli such as tax abatements, tourism and foreign investment which may not have staying power. As new glass and steel towers have risen in Manhattan, the outer boroughs have fallen into decay and burned. The magnitude of building abandonment and arson is truly staggering.

The trend of housing unit abandonment by landlords began in the 1960's. During the latter part of that decade, approximately 20,000 units were being abandoned annually.[17] By the late 1970's, this number had risen to 25,000 annually. In 1979, this translated into 150,000 apartments with a population of half a million.[18] Abandoned buildings legally became IN REM properties and are the city's responsibility. Those abandoned by landlords, may not necessarily be abandoned by tenants, meaning that the city has gradually become the principal landlord in many inner city poverty areas. In addition, these properties no longer produce real estate tax revenue for the city.

Arson and abandonment of housing units are not random events. They have their origins in public policies, specifically rent control and rent stabilization laws, demographic changes and years of underinvestment.[19] One or a combination of these forces acted in various parts of the city to create bombed out landscapes of vandalized or arsoned buildings. In the South Bronx, for example, Morris claims that housing abandonment was related to the economics of obsolete housing stock.[20] This area was densely populated from the 1920's through the 1950's and consisted of five and six story walkup tenements. As an upwardly mobile population moved out, landlords were unable to rent out the top most floors even at prices just sufficient to cover maintenance. Arson became a convenient and in some cases the only financial alternative for landlords.[21] Morris' conclusion is certainly arguable. Others would point out that rent control and rent stabilization laws made it impossible for landlords to obtain rents that would even cover the costs of routine maintenance much less capital improvements. In effect, landlords were made to subsidize tenants to a degree where income for profits, capital improvements and finally routine maintenance ceased to exist.

One of the first signs of imminent housing abandonment was an increase in real estate tax delinquencies. Because the city had a four year long foreclosure procedure, many thought non-payment was a landlord device for keeping tax money for four years in order to invest it and earn income at the city's expense. This theory was shattered when the city moved to a one year foreclosure procedure in 1976 and rapidly found itself the landlord of 30,000 housing units. The failure of landlords to pay taxes reflected the fact that the buildings were no longer worth keeping.

With the rising cost of fuel, the problem of arson and abandonment progressively became worse. But attempts on the part of political leaders to change rent control and rent stabilization laws were undertaken with hesitation and extreme caution. For the majority of voters in the city are tenants with whom such changes would be extremely unpopular. Landlords in a number of areas of the city, particularly Manhattan, have gotten around the rent control and rent stabilization laws by converting their units to cooperative apartments or condominiums.

SOCIAL PROBLEMS AND CRIME

Like all major cities in America, New York has a number of pressing social problems which escalate each year. The roots of many of these problems lie in high rates of unemployment among minority groups, such as black youths, grinding poverty and the inability of many of the city's more recent immigrants to move into the economic and social mainstream of American life. One out of every seven New Yorkers is on welfare, representing a population of 930,000.[22] In addition there are anywhere from 500,000 to 1.5 million illegal aliens in the city, most of whom are poor, uncounted and untaxed, but who avail themselves of a variety of free social and medical services.

In 1978, Senator Edward Kennedy, in addressing the 23rd annual NAACP dinner, warned of the development of a permanent underclass in many of America's cities. He cited statistics for New York City which did not take public health officials by surprise. Fifty percent of all New York blacks were born out of wedlock. This compared to 20 percent in 1956. Similarly, 30 percent of hispanics were born to mothers without husbands, compared to 11 percent in 1956.[23] These data are of significance not least of all because such a large proportion of the welfare roles are comprised of such mothers and children. They speak for societal disorganization and the emergence of a generation which is disadvantaged from the outset. They are also a manifestation of a broader social problem, that of the permanent underclass referred to by Senator Kennedy. Ill equipped for the few white collar jobs available, the poor from the inner city poverty areas cannot integrate themselves into the city's job market. And the unskilled or semi-skilled positions for which they are qualified have long since disappeared.

By the late 1970's crime had spread throughout the city, even to mid-town Manhattan where assaults on persons had been rare in the early part of the decade. But New York City did not lead the nation in various categories of crime. According to the *Uniform Crime Report* published by the Federal Bureau of Investigation, New York ranked twelfth in murders, eighteenth in forcible rape, third in assaults and second in robbery.[24] It is the latter two types of crime which are of overwhelming concern to many people, precisely because of their relatively high incidence. Crime is significantly related to drug use since a number of addicts must spend up to several hundred dollars a day to support their habits. There were approximately 150,000 individuals in drug treatment programs in the city during the 1970's and an equal number of addicts who were not receiving treatment of any kind.[25] It is difficult to determine what proportion of crime is drug related. But clearly, based on the number of addicts in the city and their daily monetary needs, it is significant. As in many other areas of the country, increasingly more crime was attributable to juvenile offenders from all socio-economic classes and the widespread availability of handguns. These trends were met in the late 1970's by legislation in New York State lowering the age limit at which juveniles could be tried as adults and by a stiff gun control law in New York City.

Auletta succinctly summed up New York City's social and crime problems when he said that the city has too many poor, too few middle class people, spreading segregation, eroding neighborhoods, youth gangs and a haunting fear of crime.[26] This certainly portays a bleak picture, but it is hardly one that can be denied. Yet, one must place it into perspective. Prior to World War I, Irish slums, for example, were characterized by fatherless families, precocious sexual amorality among children and an appalling crime rate. Such historical patterns are easily forgotten, leading to a perception of the present as unique.

POLITICAL EVENTS

Prior to the 1960s, urban politics in New York City often had a parochial focus of little national concern. Politicians came from the majority ethnic groups, the Germans, Irish, Italians, and Jews. The prevailing perception of many of them was that they were petty power brokers of low repute whose public policies were strongly influenced by a flock of interest groups that included realtors, building contractors, businessmen, and insurance agents. New York City politics tended to absorb more than its share of hack lawyers who, as judges and commissioners, doled out patronage and kept the city running on back-room deals.

The excellence that emerged from the city's ethnic immigrants tended to move into the private sector, to Wall Street law firms, midtown advertising, banking, and careers outside the city. While they concerned themselves with broader universal issues such as foreign affairs, the emerging third world, east-west relations, and pollution, the politicians continued to hone down on minutiae, besting even the ward bosses of an earlier generation. True, there were bright lights in city government now and then, and departments such as health and also hospitals that had long histories of professional leadership. But in the main, the lacklusters ran the city's affairs.

To a certain degree, this came to an abrupt end in New York City in the 1960s. What brought this change about was not merely the electoral process, but also a mounting urban crisis that had been in the making for several years. It was not only that the old tried and tested political methods were no longer working, but also that the civil rights movement in the cities spotlighted urban problems and, in so doing, moved them to the political front burner. In effect, the crisis in America's cities became the dominant domestic political issue of the decade. The quality people who had traditionally shunned local public office because of its disrepute now enthusiastically rushed into city government. An atmosphere for reform had been created by a failure of the old political methods to solve ever-mounting problems. Bereft of no option but benign neglect, the old political guard was only too happy to retreat to a safe corner and let the reformers handle the racially charged problems of the city. The reformers, for their part, were confident that the problems could be solved. All that was needed was ingenuity and determination.

This reform movement in New York City became the liberal experiment of John V. Lindsay's first mayoral term, which began in 1966.[27] The city Lindsay inherited in 1966 had been characterized by the press as a "city in crisis," although from the vantage point of the early 1980s, its problems were really only just beginning.[28] During the previous twelve years, Robert Wagner had been mayor. He brought to the office years of experience as a state assemblyman, tax commissioner, commissioner of housing and buildings, chairman of the City Planning Commission, and borough president of Manhattan. In view of Wagner's broad experience in housing, it is not surprising that his three terms as mayor witnessed major efforts to eliminate substandard housing and the construction of tens of thousands of new units. Wagner also built hundreds of schools, libraries, playgrounds, community centers, and five new hospitals. A good deal of this building had the direct imprint of Robert Moses, chairman of the Slum Clearance Committee and a member of the City Planning Commission.

Mortar and stone, however, were inadequate remedies for the city's growing ills, and Wagner knew it. Cognizant of the problems of the black and hispanic poor, he attempted to direct increasingly higher levels of city services to them.[29] He created the Attack on Poverty program in 1964, a forerunner of the national Economic Opportunity Act programs. But he did not possess the flexibility to deal with the ever-growing demands of a militant black leadership steeled from its experiences in Mississippi and Alabama. What was emerging was a confluence of the civil rights movement, now transported to New York, and the eruption of civil disorder born of years of frustration with life in the ghettos. Explosive rioting was almost inevitable; it finally broke out in Harlem and Queens in 1963. The following year, more widespread rioting broke out in Bedford-Stuyvesant and Harlem on the heels of the killing of a black youth by an off-duty police officer.[30]

Even Wagner's political adversaries had to admit frankly that he was honest and well-intentioned and that he had an impressive list of achievements that marked his tenure as mayor. But the political genius which had served him so well in the 1950s was inadequate to deal with the problems of the 1960s. In large measure, this was due not to a lack of skills on his part, but to their being mismatched with the city's growing new problems of poverty, racial polarization, crime, and deficit spending.[31] Wagner's public image suffered, as Morris has observed.[32] His subtle political instincts came across as Machiavellian, his sense of timing appeared as indolence, and his skill as a compromiser made him look like a doubletalker.[33]

Lindsay assumed office in 1966 after winning on the Republican ticket with Liberal party support. A patrician, Anglo-Saxon Protestant, he had previously served in Congress, where he had earned a reputation as a civil libertarian.[34] He was genuinely concerned with improving the lot of the poor, which in New York City meant tackling the thorny issues of housing, unemployment, education, and crime. The advantages he had over Wagner were not merely those of style but, more important, he beame mayor at a time when the national mood was swinging toward reform. In 1966 the liberals controlled Congress and President Johnson's Great Society programs were moving into high gear. Unlike Wagner, Lindsay was in a position to preside over such sweeping federal social initiatives as the Model Cities program, Medicare, Medicaid, the War on Poverty, and education reform. An expansionist mood also prevailed in the state government under the governorship of the late Nelson Rockefeller.

Lindsay walked the city streets to abort racial unrest. But in the final analysis, it was the avalanche of federal anti-poverty programs, coupled with black and hispanic control of them, which defused the ghetto anger and frustration that might otherwise have erupted into rioting. The new mayor reorganized city government, creating ten superagencies to coordinate the activities and services of city departments. He recruited hundreds of new bright and young people to serve in management positions. Armed with little other than arrogance and inexperience, many of these young people had little to recommend them besides loyalty to the mayor and dues payments as campaign workers. But there were also talented and experienced young managers who did bring about major improvements in the city's bureaucratic form and functions.

Lindsay's first term as mayor witnessed unprecedented growth in city spending. In his first two years in office, city expenditures rose by 47 percent, at a time when inflation was negligible.[35] Much of this added spending was accounted for by an increase in welfare case loads, medicaid, and labor costs. City labor unions made enormous demands on Lindsay and came away with lucrative settlements.

There were strikes of transit workers, nurses and doctors in city clinics, sanitation workers, and teachers.[36] All of these groups demanded and got large pay increases, plus added pension and other fringe benefits. These settlements would cost the city dearly in the future and would significantly contribute to the fiscal crisis of 1975.

In 1969, Lindsay's first term drew to a close. It was characterized by a philosophical commitment to social and welfare reform and, in practical terms, resulted in an enormous increase in city expenditures, gaining for the city the reputation as the welfare capital of the country. It is easy to find fault in retrospect, but one should remember that the expensive reforms that took place in New York City were not parochial. They were simply local reflections of national trends. The same holds true for employee salary and benefit package agreements. Some have cogently argued that Lindsay presided over this local manifestation of a national phenomenon.[37] But it must also be remembered that philosophically, he championed it.

Lindsay's second term (1970 to 1974) was in marked contrast to his first. The limits of expansion were realized but were not translated into action, primarily because of the mayor's preoccupation with his presidential bid. There were few new initiatives, but the momentum of earlier ones carried forward unchecked, escalating the city's debt. Budget gaps grew progressively, from $200 million in 1971 to 1972 to $800 million in 1972 to 1973, in spite of heavy borrowing and a range of financial gimmicks. To Lindsay's credit, he did achieve significant managerial reforms after he had abandoned his presidential bid in 1972. But this occurred primarily in 1973, after almost three years of diversion to national politics.

Abraham D. Beame's election in 1973 in one sense represented a desire of the electorate to return to traditional New York City politics and simpler times. Beame had previously served in the city's budget bureau and had won elective office as a Democrat for two terms as city comptroller. The dominant issue of the Beame four-year mayoralty was the fiscal crisis, which unfolded in 1974 and became full blown in the spring of 1975. It was difficult to estimate the precise magnitude of the city's operating deficit because of the use of a variety of financial and accounting gimmicks. Beame estimated it to be $450 million in late 1974, but others thought it more on the order of $630 million.[38] Postponement of dealing with the city's mounting debt was achieved through borrowing. In November 1974 alone, the city borrowed $2.5 billion, and for all of calendar year 1974 the total amount borrowed was a staggering $8.0 billion! At the same time, Fitch Investors' Service downgraded the city's bonds from a rating of A to tripe or double B according to their maturity dates.[39] Early 1975 witnessed a series of events which eventually brought matters to crisis proportions. Morris had presented a detailed chronology of these events, which included the city's inability to refinance debt to pay off maturing notes and meet operating expenses.[40] The banks, which had sizeable investments in city notes and bonds, were understandably anxious about what they perceived as a steadily deteriorating situation.

Under the impetus of the newly elected governor, Hugh Carey, the state established the Municipal Assistance Corporation (MAC) to restructure the city's debt. Its principal goal was to issue long-term bonds and use the proceeds to purchase the city's short-term notes. The MAC demanded, and got, austerity measures from Beame, including layoffs, a wage freeze, a transit fare increase, and funding cutbacks for the City University system. By August 1975, MAC had refinanced a billion dollars of the city's debt. However, there was another billion to be refinanced in September. The first wave of refinancing by MAC had included the use of pension funds and the assistance of the banks. The former could not purchase any more of the debt, and the banks were unwilling to. Additionally, the federal government refused to help.

Governor Carey then intervened, called a special session of the legislature, and proposed the creation of the Emergency Financial Control Board. The creation of this board, a majority of whose members were in the governor's camp, effectively moved fiscal management from the mayor's control. The following month, October, saw MAC bonds tumble in value. The city was now seriously close to default. Carey launched an all-out effort for federal assistance. But President Gerald Ford, then running against Jimmy Carter for the presidency, saw political liabilities attached to any aid to New York City. The *New York Daily News* carried Ford's reply in an earthy headline: "Ford to City: Drop Dead." New York City and state shortly rewarded Ford's animosity by delivering their electoral votes to Jimmy Carter, without which the presidential election would have gone to Ford.

Carey continued to pressure Washington, and a special session of the legislature passed a bill placing a three-year moratorium on the principal payments of $2.4 billion in city notes. This was an attempt to force noteholders to exchange their notes for MAC bonds. Again, the pension funds purchased a sizeable portion of the city's debt, this time $2.7 billion's worth, and the banks exchanged about a billion in notes for MAC bonds. Congress then finally enacted the Seasonal Financing Act, which gave the city $2.3 billion per annum for three years at the low rate of 1 percent. But even this did not provide a permanent solution to the city's debt problems. Once the 1975 three-year program ended, the city again faced default. But the Governor, with MAC chairman Felix Rohatyn, devised a new four-year program to balance the city's books by 1982. Its essential ingredients included federal loan guarantees, pension fund purchase of a ceiling of $1.65 billion in federally guaranteed city debt, and the purchase by banks, pension funds, and other institutions of $1.8 billion in MAC debt.[41]

In spite of these herculean efforts, substantial deficits were still projected for the remaining period of the four-year plan: $431 billion (1979 to 1980), $877 billion (1980 to 1981), and $1.16 billion (1981 to 1982). However, all of these efforts resulted in radical changes in the city's financial management systems, the refinancing or discharging of almost $4.5 billion in short-term debt, a 20 percent reduction in city employees, and a standardization of pension plans for new employees.[42]

Edward Koch, who successfully opposed Beame for the mayoralty in 1977, essentially presided over the enactment of the myriad of measures devised earlier by the Emergency Financial Control Board and the Municipal Assistance Corporation. In 1981, he was reelected mayor with bipartisan Democratic and Republican support. A deft politician endowed with a comedian's skills, he projected a dazzling popularist style that was pressed into service as a psychological tonic for a problem-wearied citizenry. But in substance, Koch was unable to reverse the city's general decline. As *The New York Times* maintained in editorials, essentially he led the public into accepting a necessary deterioration of city services.[43] Yet he himself claimed that he turned the city's affairs around after taking office in 1978.[44] Serious students of the city's affairs, however, disagreed with this self-assessment and saw little difference in Koch's spending priorities from those of Mayor Beame.[45]

To Koch's credit, he moved the mayoralty back into the center of the political stage in New York City. And he was clearly a concerned, dedicated, and sincere mayor, making the best of very difficult economic, social, and political situations. The reality that he faced was a rather grim one, characterized by a severe retrenchment of basic city services, progressive deterioration of the city's mass transit system, vandalized parks, rampant crime and unsafe streets, declining quality in public education, poor sanitation services, and a progressive atrophy of economic strength. None of these were the doing of any single mayor. Rather, they were the price that New York City paid for its good intentions.[46]

Chapter 2

THE EARLY HISTORY
OF THE NEW YORK CITY
DEPARTMENT OF HEALTH

The New York City Department of Health is the largest local health department in the U.S., and surpasses many state departments in terms of function, staffing, and budgeting. During the 1970s, this department had a staff of about 4,500 and an annual operating budget of $120 million. It performed numerous standard-setting and regulatory functions as well as delivering a variety of direct services from its central office, fifteen district health centers, seventy child health stations, and a thousand school clinics.

The department has had a long and complex history and has served as a model for many health departments around the country. It has experienced both periods of excellence and periods of decline, which have often been determined by a variety of factors, including the quality of full-time personnel, mayoral support of public health issues and programs, and the challenges of the times. The department's history has been carefully reviewed by a number of authors.[1-5] It can be argued that much of an agency's past history has little bearing on the present and, hence, there is not much point in reviewing it. This argument, however, is less convincing in light of the fact that many of the department's structures and functions have their roots in the past century and often represent not merely modern derivatives, but rather units and activities that are as relevant today as they were a century ago. It is useful therefore to take a brief look at the department's administrative history.

EARLY YEARS (1657 to 1865)

Public health problems have existed in New York since the city's founding in the seventeenth century, and probably well before when the only inhabitants of Manhattan were migratory bands of Indians. Early efforts of the Dutch, then the British, and finally the Americans to deal with these problems were sporadic and inadequate. The earliest organized public health activity was an ordinance in 1657 that prohibited people from throwing garbage and refuse in the streets.[6] This attempt by the Dutch governor, Peter Stuyvesant, was the first round of a still unsuccessful effort not only to keep the streets clean, but also to clear up the environment. At about the same time, attempts were also made to regulate slaughter houses, with varying degrees of success. It was not until 1689 that occasional quarantine orders were issued, and not until 1755 that the first quarantine law was passed.[7]

Baumgartner has cogently pointed out that for a two-hundred-year period following the late seventeenth century the twin concerns of public health officials were sanitation and the control of communicable diseases.[8] Epidemic diseases such as cholera and yellow fever devastated the city's population at unpredictable intervals, and endemic problems such as typhoid fever and tuberculosis produced a high mortality rate. These and other diseases were poorly understood, and it was not until the early part of the nineteenth century that physicians and others began theorizing about their causes and the nature of their spread. They would do so for almost a century, until the dawn of the great bacteriologic discoveries of the 1880s. Meanwhile, public health efforts often faltered, but were sometimes brilliant considering the state of knowledge at the time. They were based for the most part on a mixture of empirical observation, supposition, and theory. Understandably, they were not always successful or useful. But they did constitute a steady, if slow, progress.

As the city grew in size and complexity, it became clear that public health problems could not be dealt with by periodic ordinances. Thus, in 1784 the New York State government appointed a Health Officer of the Port, whose chief concern was the enforcement of quarantine measures.[9] The state governor, however, laid down the rules under which this health official was to function. In contrast to what had occurred over the previous hundred years, public health activities developed quickly. The first death records were filed in 1795, and reports of infectious diseases were required of physicians in 1796. That same year, the legislature empowered the city's Common Council, the chief institution of municipal government, to pass ordinances governing sanitation. A Health Office Commission composed of seven men was also appointed to administer quarantine regulations.[10]

What then evolved administratively was an assortment of positions dealing with public health matters, which were loosely coordinated. The administrative structure in 1799 consisted of a Health Office Commission, reduced from its original seven men to three. The three were the Health Officer of the Port, who dealt with quarantine, the Resident Physician, who looked for epidemic disease in the city, and the Health Commissioner who, as Blake has remarked, was, despite his title, merely an assistant to the Resident Physician.[11] All of these officials were appointed by the state, and when acting together as the Health Office Commission regulated quarantine and administered the hospital on Staten Island.

Further administrative development was, in effect, a response to the prevailing theory that yellow fever, which appeared in devastating epidemic form in 1798, was linked to filth. This theory had first been put forth in 1795 by Dr. Richard Bayley, then the Health Officer of the Port.[12] Of interest is the fact that his daughter was Saint Elizabeth Seton, founder of the Sisters of Charity of St. Vincent de Paul. Bayley was one of the city's most prominent physicians at the time.

A broad inquiry into the 1798 yellow fever epidemic was launched by the Common Council, which appointed a committee composed of its own membership and representatives from the Chamber of Commerce, the Medical Society, and the Health Office Commission. They recommended that the Common Council hire paid inspectors to levy fines against those violating sanitary ordinances. In 1796, the Common Council passed ordinances that required filling in low lots, cleansing streets, yards, and cellars, regulating noxious trades, and removing offensive and putrid goods.[13] This was in response to Bayley's recommendations.[14]

The legislature empowered the Common Council to appoint lot inspectors; from them stemmed the position of City Inspector, which was created in 1804.[15] The City Inspector was, in effect, the forerunner of the Commissioner of Health. In 1805, the legislature empowered the Common Council to appoint a Board of Health, to consist of three state selected commissioners and such others as the Council thought proper.[16]

The administrative structures that remained in place from 1805 through 1865 included the Board of Health, the Health Office Commission, and the City Inspector's Department. There were, however, some important modifications. Health wardens were appointed in 1820 by the mayor and the Common Council to inspect houses, lots, and other places. In 1823, the three Health Commissioners who had previously served ex-officio on the Board of Health were eliminated. These three, the Health Officer of the Port, the Commissioner of Health, and the Resident Physician continued their usual functions.

Needless to say, this multiplicity of positions and boards constituted an administrative nightmare and led to a considerable overlap of functions, as well as bureaucratic friction. In an attempt to reform the structure, the legislature, in 1849, sanctioned the designation of the City Inspector's office as an executive city department whose holder would be elected for a three-year term. The following year another change was implemented. It designated the mayor and the members of the Common Council as members of the Board of Health.[17] Additionally, the president of the Board of Aldermen, the president of the Board of Assistant Aldermen, the Health Officer of the Port, Resident Physician, and Health Commissioner were all designated as Health Commissioners charged with advising the mayor and the Board of Health. The Health Officer of the Port was still appointed by the governor, but the Resident Physician and the Health Commissioner became city appointees.[18] It is arguable that these administrative changes resulted in a more efficient structure. They did, however, give elected politicians a firm control over public health matters, and relegated professionals to the background.

The City Inspector's office eventually evolved to include a Bureau of Statistics and a Bureau of Sanitary Inspection, two units still in existence in the New York City Department of Health. Most of the day-to-day activities of the City Inspector revolved around sanitary problems concerning streets, vacant lots, privies, refuse, and noxious trades. Based on the *Annual Reports* of most of those who held the office, they appear to have been conscientious and dedicated. Unfortunately, they had no power to enforce the sanitary ordinances because that power was held by the Common Council. The Board of

Health acted only during times of epidemics; it was otherwise generally inactive. It was possible for City Inspectors to register gains during epidemics because of public pressure. But otherwise, the upper
hand was held by vested interest groups whose profits were linked to a
violation of sanitary regulations and who exerted enormous influence
over the politicians.

By 1850, a number of separate events were laying the foundation
for a radical change in the organization of public health services in the
city. As Duffy notes, the mid-nineteenth century witnessed an almost
total breakdown of municipal government in New York City.[19] The
roots of this breakdown were numerous. Prominent among them was
the rise of corrupt political machines, which protected the vested
interests of the few and powerful to the detriment of most. This took
place at a time when waves of Irish and German immigrants were
flowing into the city's already crowded and miserable slums.[20] Local
political bosses were able to buy immigrant support with petty favors,
while simultaneously turning their backs on the immigrants' major
problems. Year after year, City Inspectors described the terrible
conditions of filth, overcrowding, contaminated milk, crime, and
misery in the slums. The Common Council, which also constituted
the Board of Health, generally ignored their calls for action because
they were indebted to powerful interests.[21] Yet, by the 1850's, time
was running out not only for the politicians who took this approach,
but also for the wealthy few who profited from it.

A wave of social and sanitary reform swept England in the 1840s
and had a significant impact in the United States. In 1842, Sir Edwin
Chadwick published his book, *Sanitary Conditions of the Labouring
Population of Great Britain*, which became a bible for sanitary
reformers. Thomas Percival investigated fever, John Howard prisons
and hospitals, and others the Poor Laws. In 1845, John H. Griscom,
who had held the post of City Inspector from 1842 to 1843, published
a spin-off pamphlet from Chadwick's work. It was entitled *The Sanitary Conditions of the Laboring Population of New York with Suggestions for its
Improvement*.

Griscom was not the only one calling for reform. In 1843, a
group of New Yorkers formed the Association for Improving the
Condition of the Poor. They, along with the New York Academy of
Medicine and private individuals including Dr. Stephen Smith, Peter
Cooper, a merchant, William Cullen Bryant, a poet and editor of the

New York Evening Post, and Dorman B. Eaton, an attorney, began agitating for public health reform. This movement grew and attracted an increasing number of influential people, many of whom had become aware not only of the vile conditions under which the poor lived, but also of the threat of these conditions to the quality of their own lives. In 1859, the Sanitary Association of New York was formed and added its voice to the call for reform. The New York Academy of Medicine had been putting pressure on the state legislature since 1856. Other groups joined it, including the Citizens Association which, under the leadership of Stephen Smith and Dorman B. Eaton, undertook a sanitary suvey of the tenement district. The City Inspector and an alliance of Tammany Hall Democrats and upstate Republicans tried to block the pressures on the legislature for reform. But, aided by an impending cholera epidemic and the support of the press, the reformers won. In 1866, a new administrative structure for the city was set up by the state legislature. Part of this reform included the creation of the Metropolitan Sanitary District and the Metropolitan Board of Health.

THE METROPOLITAN BOARD OF HEALTH (1866 to 1870)

When the Metropolitan Board of Health was created, the city had about a million inhabitants. The new Board consisted of four health commissioners, three of whom were physicians, including the Health Officer of the Port and four police commissioners. The linking of health and police is understandable in view of the fact that at the time so many public health activities involved police action. The new health district was coterminous with the Metropolitan Police District established in 1857, and with approximately the same limits as the city has today.[22] All of the commissioners on the board were appointed by the governor, since the aim of the reform was to take public health out of Tammany Hall's control.

The new Board, subscribing to the theory that cholera was transmitted through the evacuations of patients, successfully brought under control an epidemic that had recently appeared. As a result, the Board earned enormous respect. In addition, in its first nine months of operation the board issued 22,592 orders to abate nuisances and 5,325 others giving the offenders an opportunity to request a hearing. Ashes, garbage, and rubbish were removed, yards and alleys cleaned, and many graded and paved. Bone, offal, and fat-rendering establishments were either closed or compelled to operate without allowing offensive odors to escape. Tenements were repaired and cleaned and their privies or water closets connected to sewers.[23] These were not the only accomplishments of the Board. It concerned itself with the city's milk supply and ended the use of "swill-milk," milk obtained from cows fed on brewery refuse, in Manhattan. This was such a lucrative business that swill milk dairies were maintained in conjunction with breweries.[24] The Board, however, was unable to do away with swill milk dairies in Brooklyn or to have much of an impact on street cleaning in either Manhattan or Brooklyn. The Tweed ring let out ten-year contracts in 1865 for removing garbage, ashes, offal, and dead animals from the street. These contracts were profitable for everyone except the citizens who had to live with dirty streets. In Brooklyn, the Common Council let out similar contracts.

The Board, under the direction of Charles F. Chandler, Professor of Chemistry at Columbia University, investigated the city's water and food supplies as well. The reporting of diseases by physicians was extended to include cholera, typhus, typhoid, smallpox, scarlet fever, diptheria, and measles. All reported cases were investigated, hospitalized when necessary, and disinfection emphasized as a means of control.[25] The board looked into and corrected conditions in schools, foundling asylums, and nurseries and dealt with problems as diverse as the quality of cosmetics and meat and the safety of kerosene lamps.

There were two operative divisions subordinate to the Board, the Sanitary Bureau and the Bureau of Vital Statistics. The former was headed by a physician who supervised fifteen sanitary inspectors and, eventually, several assistant sanitary inspectors. The latter was headed by a registrar. In addition, there were four other operational officers of the Board, a secretary, counsel, attorney, and engineer.[26]

Blake succinctly and eloquently summarized the record of the Metropolitan Board of Health by saying that it set high standards for energy, scientific talent, vision, and scope.[27] The Board demonstrated what could be accomplished when people concerned about public health were freed from the control of corrupt politicians. The advances that it made in four years outmatched what had been done in the previous half century. Never before had such a frontal assault been waged on the enormous sanitary and health problems of Greater New York. But in doing this, the Board had also eroded the profits of slum landlords, nuisance trades owners, and had even irritated the medical profession, which resented having to report contagious diseases and other vital data.[28]

The Board enjoyed the support of the lower socioeconomic groups who benefited from its actions and that of the upper and middle classes who found appeal in its honesty, efficiency, and success. Sustaining it further was the impression that it had successfully prevented cholera from entering the city via Europe, although it is debatable that this was the case.[29] But because the Board was an integral part of a reform movement, it was almost inevitable that it would be short lived. Once deplorable sanitary conditions had been corrected, people quickly forgot them and began focusing on the costs and inconvenience of public health measures. In a sense, the Board's successes undermined its position.[30] Additionally, the rampant political abuses associated with public health prior to the Board's creation quickly receded in people's memories once they had been abolished. But this loss of support—as soon as the glamor wore off—did not lead to the abolition of the Metropolitan Board of Health. What did was Tweed's gaining control of both the city and state democratic machines in 1869. With enough votes in the legislature, he was able to obtain a new city charter that replaced the reforms of 1866. According to Blake, this new "Tweed charter" was specifically designed to make it easier to loot the city.[31]

ESTABLISHMENT OF THE NEW YORK CITY DEPARTMENT OF HEALTH (1870 TO 1886)

The "Tweed charter" established a new Board of Health and a Department of Health. The former was composed of four police commissioners, the Health Officer of the Port, and four health commissioners appointed for five-year terms. The new department was composed of four bureaus, Sanitary Inspection, Records, Street-Cleaning, and Sanitary Permits. After Tweed fell from power in 1873, a new city charter was adopted, and the Department of Health was reduced to two bureaus, Sanitary Inspection and Vital Statistics. The Board of Health was also reduced in size to two health commissioners, the Health Officer of the Port, and the President of the Board of Police.[32]

The early years of the new Department of Health were undistinguished, not because of the influence of Tweed's political machine, which was small, but because of the severe economic depression that began in 1873. The President of the new Board of Health, Dr. Charles F. Chandler, had been professor of chemistry at Columbia University. As Duffy states, Chandler was able and honest, but was caught between fiscal retrenchment on one side and public apathy on the other. Because of the economic depression, there were the expected cries for cutbacks in city government spending. Thus, the Department of Health barely survived. In view of this, it is amazing that so much was accomplished during Chandler's ten-year tenure as President of the Board of Health. It has been argued that Chandler was not aggressive enough to prevent the relegation of public health to minor significance in the city's list of priorities.[33] But he and his small staff did make steady progress. And the department was relatively free of political interference. Blake summarized this period as one of gradual growth, rather than innovation.[34] Duffy points out that after Tweed's fall in 1873, Tammany's new leader, Honest John Kelly, allied himself with pragmatic business interests, which viewed public health as primarily benefiting the poor. As soon as cholera was no longer a serious threat, the Department of Health, although viewed as necessary, was given a low priority in city government.[35] To some extent, the Board of Health and the Department benefited from the election of a reform mayor in 1873. But reform movements usually do not have staying power, and this one was no exception.

Chandler was removed from office in 1883. He was replaced by General Alexander Shaler, who allegedly obtained the position of President of the Board of Health after promising to make the mayor's son, Dr. Cyrus Edson, the chief sanitary inspector. With Shaler in charge, the department was politicized and underwent a gradual decline. The public, however, as well as citizens groups and the press, rapidly protested the department's poor performance under Shaler. Among other things, Shaler failed to enforce sanitary laws concerning tenement houses, stated that piles of manure were not necessarily unhealthful, and was accused of suppressing reports of communicable diseases.[36] During Shaler's tenure, the department's operating budget was drastically reduced, making it difficult both for him and for the department to perform. Duffy is of the opinion that the reduction of the department's 1886 budget was a direct attack on Shaler, who clung to office in spite of criticism from the press and citizens groups and the growing suspicion of departmental corruption.[37] Shaler was arrested on December 1, 1885, for accepting a $9,000 bribe.[38] The bribe, however, had nothing to do with Shaler's Board of Health activities. It was offered by Monmouth B. Wilson, a friend who agreed to pay off a $9,000 mortgage Shaler owed on some New Jersey property. In return, Shaler, a member of the New York City Armory Board, was to recommend sites for armory construction, in which Wilson had an interest. Shaler was defended by some of New York's ablest lawyers, including Elihu Root. Two successive trials resulted in hung juries. Shaler was forcibly removed as President of the Board of Health in 1887.[39]

A GOLDEN ERA (1887 TO 1917)

The publicity and embarrassment surrounding Shaler's arrest, trial, and dismissal had a salutory effect on the department he headed. The city's new mayor, Abram Hewitt, went out of his way to reprofessionalize the Department of Health by appointing qualified men of high integrity. The staff of the department was expanded and its administrative structure overhauled. In September 1892, under the direction of Dr. Hermann Biggs, the Board of Health created a new Division of Pathology, Bacteriology, and Disinfection. The focus of the department during the 1890s was still on sanitation and the control of communicable diseases. Because of the bacteriologic advances of the 1880s, including the development of solid media for culturing bacteria, the department's assaults on epidemic diseases met with enormous success.

Facilitating the department's assault on communicable diseases was the presence from 1893 to 1897 of a reform city administration under Mayor William L. Strong and the presence within the department of a growing cadre of medical professionals. Among the most notable of these were Hermann Biggs, who would later become Commissioner of Health of New York State and William H. Park, who for many years directed the department's laboratory services. It was the work of Biggs, Park, and others in controlling tuberculosis and diphtheria in the city that earned an international reputation for the department.

In 1897, the Greater New York City Charter was adopted and put into effect on January 1, 1898. This meant that the Department of Health was now responsible for public health services over a much greater geographic area, including Richmond, Brooklyn, and Queens.[40] At the same time, the reform government of Mayor Strong was swept out of office by Tammany's Robert A. Van Wyck. During his four-year term, the department held its own, but did not make significant progress. Duffy is of the opinion that this may have been in the department's best interest at the time. It was in the midst of extending its services and administrative structure into the newly acquired boroughs. In practical terms this meant assuming the functions of twelve boards of health in Queens and eight separate village boards in Richmond.

Mayor Van Wyck appointed Nathan Strauss as president of the Board of Health in 1898. Strauss was not only a prominent businessman, but also a philanthropist. He was already widely known for establishing milk stations around the city where the poor could obtain milk at cost or free. These stations eventually became the Child Health stations of the Department of Health.[41] Strauss resigned within a year, primarily because he ran afoul of the medical profession. He had moved to make tuberculosis and other communicable diseases reportable and had also supported the sale of vaccines and antitoxins by the department. Organized medicine opposed both. In fact, the New York County Medical Society sponsored the Brush Bill in the state senate; if it had been passed, it would have reorganized the department and satisfied the position of organized medicine.[42] Another source of friction stemmed from the fact that the city's Board of Health was dominated by laymen; this did not go over well with physicians. Organized medicine was growing in strength at this time, flexing its muscle and looking for confrontations. Thus, Strauss's successor, Michael C. Murphy, although not especially qualified for the position, showed some wisdom in having the Board of Health assume a low profile.

The department's administrative structure was changed at this time. It still consisted of two bureaus, Sanitary and Records. But the former was now divided into several divisions, namely, Sanitary Inspection, Food Inspection, Contagious Diseases, Offensive Trades, Bacteriology, Medical Inspection of Schools, and Marine Inspection. Five assistant sanitary superintendents were appointed, one for each borough, to assist with administration. The rudiments of a borough structure for public health services were thus established.

As 1901 dawned, the Board of Health was headed by another layman and political appointee, John B. Sexton, who was even less qualified than his predecessor, Michael C. Murphy. Although the Board of Health became progressively tainted with political appointees during the 1890s, the Department of Health, which it supervised, made enormous leaps forward, largely because of its staff and the great scientific discoveries of the time. In examining the accomplishments of the department during this period, one finds the institution of diphtheria antitoxin use in 1895, the requiring of permits to sell milk in 1896, compulsory reporting of tuberculosis in 1897, acquisition of the Kingston Avenue Contagious Disease Hospital in 1898, and the adoption of sanitary regulations for saloons, lodging houses, and boarding houses in 1900.[43]

In 1901, a reform government was elected under Mayor Seth Low. He appointed Dr. Ernest J. Lederle as both president of the Board of Health and Commissioner of Health. It is from this date that the title Commissioner of Health was used to mean the chief executive officer of the Department of Health. The reformers revised the city's charter and Dr. Lederle restructured the Department of Health. The department expanded in size, reflecting its increasing responsibilities and broadening scope. Included in this scope was responsibility for hospitals, especially the Willard Parker Hospital and the Kingston Avenue Hospital, where patients with communicable diseases were hospitalized. The school health program was greatly improved, and full-time physicians were employed. Overall, the department's expansion and growing administrative structure was a response geared to improving sanitation and controlling communicable diseases.

In 1903, Mayor Low's reform movement was swept out of office by Tammany Hall. The new mayor, George B. McClellan, son of the Civil War general, appointed Dr. Thomas Darlington, a private practitioner, as Commissioner of Health.[44] Darlington, despite the political origins of his appointment, performed extremely well and in close collaboration with Dr. Hermann Biggs. Winslow has noted that the Department of Health benefited from the fact that Charles F. Murphy, once president of the Board of Health (1899 to 1900), was now the head of Tammany Hall. In addition, Hermann Biggs, who maintained a private practice, had cared for Murphy when he was ill with typhoid fever. This gave Biggs access to the Tammany leadership and enabled him to obtain support for many of the Department of Health's programs.[45] But it also resulted in a hands-off policy by the politicians. It would be another fifteen years before attempts were made to politicize the department again.

The first decade of the twentieth century witnessed the continued development of strong centralized divisions in the department's two bureaus, Sanitary Inspection and Records. As these divisions grew in number and size, they often overshadowed the bureau of which they were a part. They were usually oriented toward a specific medical specialty, such as child health, and had large field organizations often operating under the direction of prominent professionals. An example was the Division of Child Hygiene, established in 1908 under Dr. S. Josephine Baker. This division had 192 medical inspectors, 195 nurses, supervisors, and administrators, and a large clerical staff.[46] Dr. Baker, an extremely dynamic woman, rapidly achieved a national reputation for her innovative approach to child health. And indeed, she is still remembered today as one of the great public health leaders of the twentieth century.

The department expanded with the city and its population, yet its organizational structure remained essentially the same, with divisions formed, grouped, and regrouped under the two bureaus. It was obvious that this structure could not function for long. In addition, it was becoming clear that a highly centralized department could not continue to deal with the growing problems of a progressively decentralizing population. Although some attempts were made at decentralization in 1898, with the appointment of borough sanitary superintendents, the forces favoring centralization continued to dominate.[47]

In 1909, Tammany beat the reformers, and William L. Gaynor was elected mayor. The department had thrived and grown under the reformers and their Commissioner of Health, Dr. Thomas Darlington. But the shift of control to Tammany did not adversely affect the department. For as Duffy points out, Tammany was aware of the political value of public health and the respect with which the public held the Department of Health.[48] And Charles Murphy, the political boss of Tammany, adopted a hands-off attitude toward the department.

Tammany's choice for Commissioner of Health was Dr. Ernest Lederle, who had previously served in the post from 1902 to 1903. At the time of Lederle's assumption of office for a second term, the department had approximately a thousand employees and an annual operating budget of a million dollars. The department continued to expand during Lederle's second term. And professionals like Dr. S. Josephine Baker found that it was often easier to work with Tammany than it had been to work with the reformers.

Mayor Gaynor died in the fall of 1913 and was succeeded by a fusion mayor, John Purroy Mitchell. He reappointed Lederle, but Lederle resigned a short time afterwards and was replaced by Dr. Sigismund T. Goldwater, who served as Commissioner of Health from 1913 to 1915. Goldwater had already achieved a reputation as an eminent hospital administrator and architect and was the superintendent of Mount Sinai Hospital at the time of his appointment. Although his tenure as head of the department was brief, Goldwater presided over the first major administrative reorganization since the department's establishment forty-five years before. Under this reorganization, which had begun under Lederle in 1913, nine bureaus were created. These included the two original bureaus, Sanitary and Records, with seven divisions of the former now elevated to bureau status. These were Food Inspection, Child Hygiene, Infectious Diseases, Laboratories, Hospitals, General Administration, and Public Health Education. The last named was set up in 1914 under Dr. Charles F. Bolduan, once an assistant sanitary inspector.[49]

Goldwater, however, sought a more profound administrative reform. He and his assistants, Dr. Haven Emerson (who would succeed him as Commissioner of Health) and Dr. Alfred E. Shipley, the department's secretary (who would later become Professor and Chairman of the Department of Preventive Medicine and Community Health at the Long Island College of Medicine) pointed out a number of deficiencies in the department's structure. They found a lack of coordination between bureaus. Bureau directors were too far removed from field activities. There was an enormous amount of duplication of function between bureaus and unevenness of performance in various areas of the city. In order to remedy these deficiencies, Goldwater, Emerson, and Shipley proposed decentralizing the department by setting up district offices under the direction of physicians who would oversee the activities of the various bureaus. These district health officers, as they were to be called, would, in effect, be mini-health commissioners. Shipley was familiar with the line and staff concept advanced by Frederick Taylor, an administration and efficiency expert who enjoyed great renown at the time. Thus,

Shipley stated that the health officer and his field staff would be responsible for line work and that the bureaus would serve in staff positions.[50]

As Kaufman points out, the bureau directors saw these proposals as a direct threat to their supremacy and status, and as potentially disruptive of the whole fabric of informal organization that had existed for a generation.[51] Thus began the long struggle between two opposing forces within the department, those favoring centralization and those favoring decentralization.[52]

The bureau directors responded to the reorganization plan in 1914 with arguments that have since been used by generations of their successors. Bureau directors were all specialists in specific fields. A district health officer could not possibly master all these specialties. Bureau directors could not be held responsible for the technical quality of work carried out by personnel reporting to a district health officer. Decentralization was scarcely required in a city with rapid mass transit where personnel could be fielded to any location in a matter of minutes. And finally, they argued that the coordination of health district activities would prove more difficult than those of bureaus.[53]

Despite these objections, Goldwater set up a pilot health district in Manhattan's Lower East Side. It was called Health District No. 1, and it became functional in November 1914. Within a year, Goldwater, Emerson, and Shipley announced that they were pleased with the results of the pilot. Local civic organizations showed an interest in building a community health program, and the department was able to deliver more services at lower cost by shifting local departmental personnel from one categorical activity to another as the need arose.[54]

On October 31, 1915, Goldwater resigned to become a private consultant in hospital management. During his brief tenure, he had presided over the most dramatic reorganization in the department's history. True, the reform nature of Mayor Mitchell's government made this reorganization possible. However, it would not have taken place without Goldwater's leadership. He was succeeded in office by Dr. Haven Emerson, who decided to extend the district health plan to the borough of Queens where he opened four new districts in 1916. Emerson's tenure was a distinguished one marked by a number of accomplishments. But what truly characterized his two-year term was both the geographic extension of the health district concept and its expansion to include more services. He established a Division of Health Districts through which district health officers reported directly to the commissioner. Bureau directors were advisors to this division and had no authority over its decisions. Emerson drew up plans for extending the idea to Brooklyn, and envisioned having forty to fifty districts of 100,000 people for the entire city.[55] These plans, however, were to be shelved for almost sixteen years.

During the 1917 election, incumbent Mayor Mitchell, a reformer, found himself in a four-way race. Prior to the election, a delegation of physicians and druggists from Brooklyn and Queens had met with Mitchell and had urged the creation of a separate department with its own health commissioner for these two boroughs. Their intent was to weaken the department because they chafed under its regulations. Tammany Hall shortly announced that if elected, it would establish a health department in each borough, each with its own commissioner. John F. Hylan, Tammany's candidate, won in the November election and took office the following January. He removed Emerson as Commissioner of Health on January 16, 1918, and appointed a Bronx surgeon, Dr. J. Lewis Amster as his successor. Amster was then president of the Bronx County Medical Society and an active Democrat. Thus ended one of the finest periods in the department's history. For Hylan was not only determined to dismantle the department, but also to politicize what remained of it and rid himself of the professionals. What ensued were eight years during which the department's professionals successfully held their own against Hylan and the Tammany politicians. But they were not merely years of travail as Duffy has characterized them, but ones of decline as well.[56]

STRUGGLE AND DECLINE (1918 TO 1925)

Although John Hylan was backed by Tammany Hall, he was primarily the candidate of William Randolph Hearst, the newspaper tycoon. Therefore, Tammany's influence over him had its limits. Hylan lost no time in making a frontal assault on the Department of Health. In April 1918, three months after assuming office, he told Amster, his Commissioner of Health, to fire seven of the department's nine bureau directors. Among them was Dr. S. Josephine Baker, the head of the Bureau of Child Hygiene. Hylan was intent on decentralizing the department and politicizing it, ends which could only be achieved by breaking up the central structure of the bureaus and stripping them of their professional leadership. In taking this course of action, he greatly underestimated the magnitude of the opposition that eventually developed, and was seemingly oblivious to the fact that most bureau directors were protected by civil service. As Duffy has noted, Hylan's actions caused an uproar of protest from the medical societies, civic groups, labor unions, and newspapers. And the protests grew even stronger when he proposed abolishing the Bureau of Child Hygiene as an economy measure.[57]

Amster initially went along with Hylan's plans, probably out of political loyalty and inexperience. Dr. Baker observed that Amster was actually bewildered by Hylan's demands.[58] On April 9, 1918, James E. McBride, the chairman of the Civil Service Commission, started secret hearings on the legal status of the bureaus. This caused an enormous uproar, which prompted Hylan to change his strategy. He now claimed that the hearings were for the purpose of investigating corruption in the Department of Health. As April moved on, Amster became extremely uncomfortable about presiding over Hylan's unpopular and destructive plans. He told the mayor that the McBride investigation was damaging the department and that the abolition of the bureaus would jeopardize the public health. McBride then issued a preliminary report and held the remaining hearings in public. Hylan then told Amster to remove Drs. Jacobi and Goldwater from the department's Medical Advisory Board.[59]

Amster was certainly willing to accommodate Hylan's political appointments at various levels in the department. But as Baker says, there came a time when he could stand it no longer. For Hylan's assault was bent on the almost total destruction of the department. Finally, on April 29, Amster resigned, as he had told Baker he would, with a strong statement denouncing Hylan's attempts to destroy the department.[60]

Hylan then appointed Dr. Royal S. Copeland as commissioner. Copeland was an eye specialist with no background in public health. He was, however, dean of the New York Homeopathic Medical College and director of Flower Hospital. A native of Michigan and a descendant of an old New England family, he was, as Duffy has so well characterized him, a shrewd politician with some interest in public welfare.[61] He was flamboyant, outspoken, and quick to support causes with broad popular appeal. He was also politically ambitious and adept at extracting every bit of political mileage from all sorts of issues, even those with only a tangential relationship to public health. He appealed to people's prejudices when he expressed alarm at the low birth rate among native mothers compared to that among the foreign born, and to women's vanity when he defended feminine silk stockings and high heels, characterizing the prevailing fashion of long skirts as conducive to catching germs from the streets.[62] He was commissioner during the great influenza pandemic of 1918, which also gave him enormous exposure in the press.

Copeland had serious political ambitions of his own, and consequently not only maintained a high public profile in the press but also accommodated Mayor Hylan's politicization program in the Department of Health. Unlike Amster, he knew how to handle Hylan, and quietly helped him deprofessionalize the department while he simultaneously projected an image as a public health crusader. Copeland effectively rode public health issues to political success. He achieved many things during his four-year tenure, but a number of them were in the service of his personal political ambition. As Duffy has noted, he fought for lower milk prices and heated tenements; he tried to deal with drug addiction, sympathized with coal strikers, and advocated public housing.[63] But he also accommodated Hylan's numerous political appointments and established borough health offices so that departmental personnel would be more cooperative with local political leaders. During his tenure, the department was deprofessionalized, a process which often went unnoticed because of his ability to shrewdly divert the press with his ephemeral crusades. In short, Copeland was politically, not professionally, oriented.[64] In September 1922, Copeland was chosen as the Democratic nominee for the United States Senate and rode to victory in November on a platform of public health issues, upsetting the Republican incumbent. Prior to leaving the department, he paved the way for Hylan's personal physician, Dr. Frank J. Monaghan, to become Commissioner of Health by appointing him a deputy commissioner.

Hylan, who had been reelected to a second four-year term in November 1921, quickly appointed Monaghan as his new Health Commissioner. He served in the post until the end of Hylan's term in December 1925. Copeland's political astuteness and quick mind enabled him to get both on-the-job training and effectively deal with the mayor, press, public, and professionals. But Monaghan simply stumbled along, with the department pretty much running on its own. It was during his tenure that Dr. S. Josephine Baker finally resigned as head of the Bureau of Child Hygiene, and that the department went into a steep decline. Although the department had begun its decline under both Amster and Copeland, it was during Monaghan's administration that the accumulated abuses became too great and too numerous to hide. In fact, by 1925, Tammany decided not to support Hylan for reelection because of the mounting evidence of widespread corruption during his two terms as mayor. It was not that Tammany was adverse to corruption, only that it had now gotten out of hand and had become both a major public issue and a political liability.

REVIVAL (1926 TO 1933)

James J. Walker was elected mayor in November 1925, replacing John Hylan. He publicly announced that the goal of his administration would be to take politics out of the Department of Health. In view of what followed, this was no mere publicity ploy. Walker actively sought the advice of the New York Academy of Medicine, the state health commissioner, and various medical societies. On January 1, 1926 he appointed Dr. Louis I. Harris as commissioner. Harris was a public health professional who was then the head of the Bureau of Preventable Diseases. Of interest is the fact that fifty-one years later, in 1977, one of his successors as head of the bureau would also be appointed Commissioner of Health.

Harris's two-fold task was to clean the department of the neglect and corruption of the previous eight years and to bring the department's activities up to date.[65] As Duffy has pointed out, there was widespread departmental malfeasance when Harris assumed office. Thomas J. Clougher, whom Copeland had appointed to the position of secretary, had been in charge of the Special Service Division, a unit also created by Copeland for dispensing Health Department permits. Clougher, who controlled the appointment of inspectors, was later indicted, tried, and finally sentenced for from five to ten years in prison for bribery.[66] He was not the only one accused of either malfeasance or bribe taking. Before the year was out, a total of twenty-six employees resigned, six quickly retired before proof of guilt could be established, and fifteen were fired after trials.[67] In order to assist Harris in cleaning up the department, Mayor Walker appointed Judge Charles M. Kelby as special counsel for the investigation.

Harris had to restructure a department whose scaler form had been altered to facilitate political patronage during the Hylan years. A number of divisions, such as the Milk Division, the Chemical Laboratory, the Veterinary Division, the Division of Industrial Hygiene, and the Otisville Sanitarium had been moved directly under the commissioner's control, where people such as Clougher dispensed patronage and accepted bribes.

In August 1927, Judge Kelby submitted a final report to Mayor Walker that documented widespread graft among food inspectors. A grand jury investigation followed, and five individuals were indicted. Many others, however, escaped prosecution by turning state's witness. Kelby also uncovered a slush fund of a million dollars that had been used between 1921 and 1925.[68]

The best summation of the department inherited by Harris was given by Charles—Edward Amory Winslow in the *New York Times*. He wrote: "Ten years ago, it was beyond question that New York City had the best municipal health department in the world. In 1918 came a change, and for the first time in thirty years the blight of political influence fell upon the splendid social machinery."[69] Harris now successfully rebuilt that machinery. He established a Bureau of Nursing and reestablished the Bureau of Health Education under Dr. Charles F. Bolduan, who had been sacked during the Hylan administration. He worked hard to bring the department's hospitals up to a Grade A standard as defined by the American College of Surgeons. He was also successful in getting a quarter of a million dollar increase in the department's budget in 1926, making a total budget of over six million dollars for fiscal year 1927

Probably no other New York City Commissioner of Health, except for Dr. Lowell E. Bellin in 1974, had to assume the enormous task of reprofessionalizing the department. Harris was eminently successful, and by 1928 the department had regained not only its former professional qualities but had also been restructured to meet the major public health issues of the day. Additionally, Harris had aned the department of wholesale graft and corruption. The New

York City Department of Health had come close to collapse, and Harris and his professional colleagues, with the support of many medical groups and the mayor, had brought it back from the brink.

On August 16, 1928, Harris stepped down as Commissioner of Health and retired after twenty years of service in the Department of Health. He was succeeded by his deputy, Dr. Shirley W. Wynne, thus setting a precedent that would be repeated several times in succeeding decades. Wynne, a public health professional, was Commissioner of Health for five and a half years. During his first few months in office, a separate Department of Hospitals was created, encompassing the hospitals that had long been administered by the Department of Health.

One of the most significant developments during Wynne's commissionership was the revival of the district health plan that had been shelved in 1918. The impetus for this revival did not come from the Department of Health, but from a number of outside groups. In fact, the idea had been taken up in 1918 by a group that set up the Mulberry Health Center. The Bowling Green Neighborhood Association had even opened a center as early as 1916. Finally, an East Harlem Health Center was established in 1921. However, the major breakthrough came in 1926 with the opening of the Bellevue-Yorkville Health Demonstration.[70] Organized in 1924, it was funded largely by the Milbank Memorial Fund. The Department of Health was formally integrated into the demonstration project and eventually assumed leadership of it by 1929. The center essentially offered a wide variety of health and social services to the people of this area situated on the east side of Manhattan. The Department of Health placed many of its traditional activities, such as tuberculosis control and a baby health station, in the demonstration, and tried out new administrative techniques there.[71]

The success of the demonstration led to Dr. Wynne's appointment of a Committee on Neighborhood Health Development, whose purpose was to be the planning of a city-wide network of health centers. On October 28, 1929, the committee presented a preliminary report in which it recommended the division of the city into thirty health districts. The committee also recommended that the city spend $ four million building sixteen centers over the succeeding four years.[72] On October 29, 1929, the stock market crashed on Wall

Street, and the Great Depression began. Only one center was opened, the Central Harlem Health Center in 1930, in rented quarters.

The dawn of 1930 witnessed a decline in tax revenues for the city, and mounting deficits and reduced departmental budgets. The Department of Health was not spared. Its budget dropped by a million dollars from the previous year. As the country's economic situation grew progressively worse, it became increasingly difficult for the department to carry out its routine functions, much less initiate any new programs. As unemployment rose, demands on the department's free services grew, yet the department's budget and staff were cut. Wynne and his staff held the department together as best they could. And in 1933, Wynne requested that the American Public Health Association evalute the department. They did so with a grant from the Commonwealth Fund and concluded that most of the department's deficiencies were due to inadequate financing.[73]

Meanwhile, larger political events unfolded with the resignation under pressure of Mayor Walker in September 1932. Walker's youthful and dapper appearance had made him an extremely popular mayor. But this popularity could not sustain him in the face of mounting suspicion of graft and corruption. After his resignation, an acting mayor, John V. McKee, was appointed. He ran the following year in the 1933 municipal elections in a three-way race, losing to the Republican candidate, Fiorello La Guardia.

The department was untouched by the scandals of the Walker administration. But La Guardia clearly did not want a holdover Commissioner of Health. Wynne thus announced his retirement on December 16, 1933. He had served as commissioner during one of the most trying and difficult times in the country's history. The Great Depression had made strategic retreats necessary and to their credit Wynne and his staff had made them without sacrificing the public health.

Chapter 3

THE RECENT HISTORY
OF THE NEW YORK CITY
DEPARTMENT OF HEALTH

The dividing line between the Department of Health's early history and its recent one is, to a certain degree, arbitrary. However, with the advent of the first LaGuardia mayoralty in 1934, the department underwent major structural reforms and was decentralized in an unprecedented manner with the establishment of health districts. A structure was put into place that would last for several decades. There were periodic modifications in both form and function to meet current public health problems. And the opposing forces of centralization and decentralization continued to do battle, with their points of view prevailing in an almost cyclical fashion. But throughout this period, the department's structure remained unchanged.

REFORM AND REORGANIZATION (1934 TO 1949)

Fiorello La Guardia was a reform mayor with a genuine interest in public health and welfare. The success of his reform measures was due not only to his own commitment to progressive public policies, but also the "New Deal" administration of President Franklin D. Roosevelt. Roosevelt's programs were directed at solving the enormous social and ecnomic problems generated during the Great

Depression that began in 1929. Among these were numerous public health programs in the form of money grants to states and localities. It was this federal action which proved to be of vital importance in the development of the Department of Health.[1]

La Guardia appointed Dr. John Levi Rice as Commissioner of the department. Rice came to New York City from New Haven, Connecticut, where he had been head of a department that had been largely responsible for the city receiving the American Public Health Association's award for the healthiest city in its class.[2] Rice remained on as Commissioner of Health for eight and a half years until his resignation in July 1942. The department he inherited had been decimated and demoralized by the Great Depression, a situation well-documented in 1933 by the American Public Health Association, which had been asked to survey the department by Commissioner Wynne. All of the department's bureaus failed to provide minimum service. The major problem was inadequate funding, but there were also problems of uneven allocations within the department. The department had lost most of its leaders. Of the ten major bureaus and divisions only three, Laboratories, Health Education, and Nursing, had full-time, qualified directors. All the others were directed by part-time or acting directors. Morale was low and there had been no pay raises in several years.[3]

Economic necessity had forced many employees to dodge work so that they could earn money outside the department. Rice brought two hundred employees upon charges for rule infractions in 1934. And, as an economy measure, he asked that those with twenty years of service or more retire voluntarily. He also agreed to a 10 percent cut in the department's budget and eliminated 436 positions.[4] In 1934, the department's budget was about $ four million.[5]

Rice first turned his attention to reorganizing the bureaus and to hiring directors with both technical skills and leadership abilities. Technical innovations were made possible, in part because of assistance from the federal Works Progress Administration (WPA). This was especially true in the Sanitary Bureau. Help also came from the federal Emergency Relief Bureau, which provided funds for a school dental program. And WPA provided monies for physicians to conduct school entry physical exams for children whose parents could not afford them. What unfolded during Rice's early tenure was a reorganization and upgrading of the department, made possible by various kinds of federal subsidies and a simultaneous reduction in city tax levy support of the department. As President Roosevelt's national recovery efforts gained momentum during the 1930s, they made available unusual resources without which the department could not have emerged from its Great Depression decline.

Although Rice brought about enormous improvements in the department's largely centralized structure, more significantly, he launched the health district plan that had been sputtering along for almost twenty years. This was made possible not only because of pressures brought about by the Committee on Neighborhood Health Development, originally appointed by Commissioner Wynne, but also because of a commitment to the idea by both Rice and LaGuardia and the availability of federal monies to support an extensive building program.[6] Rice, however, did not think that a district system could work except under a strong central departmental office. Also, he rightly perceived that the bureaus had lost a great deal of power to the Committee on Neighborhood Health Development which, over the years, had come to exert enormous influence and authority over the internal affairs of the department.[7] In order to deal with this thorny set of problems, Rice decided to strengthen the bureaus while simultaneously launching the district health plan. In 1934, he created the Bureau of District Health under Dr. Margaret W. Barnard, the former medical director of the Bellevue-Yorkville Demonstration. Seven of the thirty planned district health officers were hired, and an ambitious building program was planned with funds provided by the Public Works Administration (PWA). By December 1935, there were PWA funds to build eight new health center buildings. By 1939, nine new district health center buildings were in operation and five more were under construction.[8] In addition, federal aid made possible the construction of a new ten-story headquarters building at 125 Worth Street, which was dedicated on November 26, 1935.[9] This building, where the Department of Health is still housed, also became headquarters for the departments of Sanitation and Hospitals.

Once the health districts and their centers were functional, the problem of conflict between bureau heads and district health officers inevitably arose. In essence, field personnel now assigned to work out of district health centers were to report on technical matters to the bureau directors and on administrative matters to the district health officers. But there were frequent differences of opinion about what was technical and what was administrative, and conflicts occurred all the time. Rice resorted to a variety of administrative devices, including his own personal intervention, to reduce the frequency of these conflicts. This was less than successful because he leaned strongly toward the bureau chiefs, or at least was perceived as doing so. Rice then invited Professor Ira V. Hiscock of the Department of Public Health at Yale to study the problem and make recommendations. He suggested, after lengthy study, that the health officers and central office be brought into closer contact and that a manual on district health administration be written.[10] Such a document was prepared in draft form. It met with a cool reception and was never used. The conflict continued in the absence of any plan to work out satisfactory relationships between functional and geographic chiefs.

As Kaufman so well describes, the area and functional people learned to live with one another in a sort of intermittent and uneasy truce.[11] But as the district system grew, clashes became more frequent. Finally, in 1941, Rice took a drastic step. He abolished the position of Director of District Health Administration and ordered that district health officers take up matters relating to a bureau directly with the chief of that bureau. Dr. Barnard was appointed Consultant in Local Administration, basically a staff position with no line authority. In Kaufman's words, "the swing away from the Goldwater doctrine was almost complete."[12] What resulted was that bureau staff operated in the health centers as independent tenants, reporting directly to their chiefs at 125 Worth Street. The district health officers presided over these activities as little more than moderators with no effective control.[13]

In 1937, three years after La Guardia took office, a new city charter became effective. It contained important provisions concerning the department. The Board of Health had been the chief executive of the Department of Health since 1901. However, in 1928, the charter was amended so that the Commissioner of Health became head of the department. But the Board of Health retained a number of administrative powers. The new charter transferred these powers to the commissioner, making the Board of Health a purely legislative body that dealt with the Sanitary Code.[14]

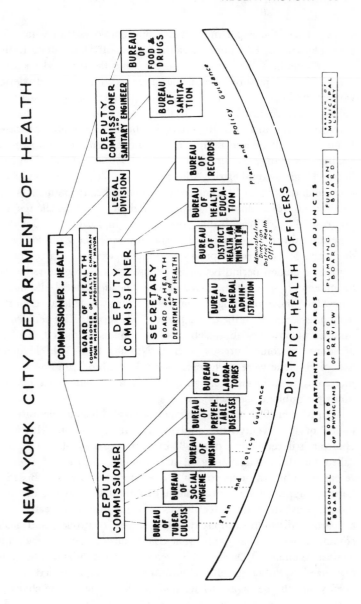

Figure 3-1 Organization chart for the New York City
Department of Health, 1939

In 1939, the department had 2,800 employees, of whom 500 were physicians, 800 public health nurses, 300 laboratory technicians, 65 dentists, 250 health inspectors, and the remainder statisticians, X-ray operators, veterinarians, accountants, and clerical workers.[15] There were twelve bureaus directing a wide variety of inspectional, regulatory, standard setting, and service activities. These bureaus included Records, Sanitary, Preventable Diseases, Laboratories, Food and Drugs, Health Education, General Administration, Nursing, Tuberculosis, Social Hygiene, Child Hygiene-School Hygiene and District Administration. The department had 15 functional district health centers and 76 child health stations. As the 1930s drew to a close, so did a period of dynamic change and progress. World War II had broken out in Europe, and federal programs aimed at rectifying the economy were being phased out as the effects of the Great Depression disappeared. The department had enjoyed a golden period because of these federal programs. District health centers were built, as well as a new headquarters building and a new laboratory building. Equally important was federal support of personnel services. In the department's 1937 report, Rice detailed the number of positions funded by federal monies. Almost half of the personnel in some bureaus such as Nursing and Child Hygiene-School Hygiene were on federal funds. WPA funds, however, were increasingly withdrawn, obliging the city to provide more tax levy funds for public health services.

In March 1941, the Department of Health held a celebration in honor of its seventy-fifth anniversary. In a speech, Mayor La Guardia (still remembered in 1981 by some departmental employees) called for the establishment of a municipal institute of scientific research within the department. A few months later the Board of Estimate approved an appropriation of $100,000 to finance the institute. In July, the Public Health Research Institute was created, with a board of directors composed of the mayor, controller, and health commissioner.[16] That same year La Guardia ran for reelection against William O'Dwyer, the Democratic candidate. The latter organized a Public Health Committee, which proceeded to levy twenty-one charges against Rice and the department. The chairman of this committee was a former departmental employee, Dr. Emanuel M. Josephson, who had been investigated for improper conduct on three occasions. And the department's personnel board had twice recommended his dismissal. Another member of O'Dwyer's committee had been found guilty of unethical conduct by the New York County Medical Society in 1928.[17] The charges were all clearly false and, as Duffy notes, the questionable character of the individuals making them nullified their effect.[18]

La Guardia was reelected in November and reappointed Rice. However, Rice's health suffered, and he resigned the following July. He had served as Commissioner of Health during a very unusual time and under a dynamic progressive mayor. This, coupled with his own dedication, honesty, and splendid abilities, resulted in an unprecedented development not only in the department's programs and functions but also in its physical plant. It was no easy matter working with La Guardia, who was forceful and who, with the finest of intentions, tended to interfere.[19] But, as Duffy notes, Rice was able to get on with La Guardia through a judicious mixture of firmness and concession.

Dr. Ernest L. Stebbins, who had been Professor of Epidemiology at Columbia University was named Commissioner of Health in July 1942. Stebbins' commissionership spanned the period of the Second World War and consequently he had to mobilize the department to meet special problems created by the war. In 1943, he attempted to resolve the conflict between the bureaus and the districts by building up the headquarters structure of district administration. He established the position of Assistant Commissioner for District Administration and appointed Dr. Margaret Barnard. She was now in a hierarchical position above those of the bureau directors and given responsibility for general supervision over and relationships between district and bureau activities.[21]

The war caused social dislocations and demands for expanded maternal and child health services. A Nutrition Division was established in 1943 and a day care unit as well. The latter concerned itself with establishing and enforcing a comprehensive set of regulations covering not only safety and hygiene in day care centers, but also physical and mental health as well. As more and more women went to work because of the war effort, the number of day care centers grew. The Emergency Maternity and Infant Care Act of 1943, which provided maternity and child care benefits for the wives and children of lower paid military personnel resulted in a grant of $6.8 million to the department. The program which resulted and which became a model for the rest of the country was designed by Dr. Leona Baumgartner, the head of the Bureau of Child Hygiene.[22]

In 1945, Stebbins was offered the position of Dean of the School of Public Health at Johns Hopkins University. La Guardia who was up for reelection did not run, and the candidate he supported, Newbold Morris, lost to the Democrat, William O'Dwyer. Stebbins agreed to stay on for several months or so until a successor could be found. O'Dwyer, who eventually resigned under a cloud of suspicion of graft and corruption before his second term was up, appointed a search committee. This committee, chaired by Dr. Thomas Parran, the Surgeon General, came up with several names. O'Dwyer, however, rejected all of them. Prior to this time, Stebbins had declared a state of imminent peril and had issued an order to shut down industry in order to conserve fuel. This was in response to a tugboat workers' strike and an emergency proclamation by O'Dwyer, who had been informed by the Office of Defense Transportation that such a strike would result in a fuel shortage. These drastic actions naturally led to enormous economic disruptions and loud protests from business and industry. Yet, as Duffy notes, Stebbins had no choice because it was February and the weather was cold and snowy. A prolonged strike would have resulted in fuel shortages.[23] Complicating the situation was a radio pronouncement by La Guardia urging Stebbins to leave the department.[24] O'Dwyer called Stebbins to City Hall and suggested he leave for Johns Hopkins the next day. Then he announced the appointment of Dr. Edward M. Bernecker as Commissioner of Health. Bernecker, who had been head of the Department of Hospitals, did not have either the legal or personal qualifications for the position. A storm of protest arose from the New York Academy of Medicine, the Board of Health, and civic groups, all of whom accused O'Dwyer of politicizing the department.[25]

O'Dwyer had to withdraw the Bernecker appointment nine days after he made it. He then chose a very obscure candidate, Dr. Israel Weinstein, director of the Bureau of Public Health Education. Duffy relates that Weinstein's appointment was greeted with a mixture of amusement and derision.[26] During the 1970s, it was still remembered in the Department of Health as an enigmatic appointment. Weinstein was a pleasant and kind man, but no great beacon of administrative ability. However, during the twenty months he served as commissioner, he did restructure the department's restaurant inspection program and successfully directed the city's efforts to prevent an outbreak of smallpox in March and April of 1947.

O'Dwyer had a lot of second thoughts about Weinstein's appointment, to the extent that when he addressed the annual meeting of the American Public Health Association in New York City he admitted that he had learned a lot about public health since taking office. He gently dismissed Weinstein and then appointed Dr. Harry I. Mustard, then the Director of the Columbia University School of Public Health. He assumed office on November 4, 1947, and remained until December 31, 1948, when he left to take a position with the State Charities Aid Association.

Although Mustard's tenure was short, it was characterized by a number of major organizational changes in the department. He was determined to resolve the conflicts between the central bureaus and the districts. In this he was assisted by a record blizzard that dumped twenty-six inches of snow on the city the day after Christmas 1947. The department was bombarded by thousands of calls from people asking for all kinds of help. Mustard found that his staff in the districts kept referring back to central headquarters for instructions instead of initiating action at the local level.[27]

On January 1, 1948, the issued a drastic four-point program. First, the district health officer was made responsible for all the localized activities of the Department of Health. Second, all communications, even technical ones from bureau chiefs to field staff, had to pass through the office of the Director of District Health Administration. Third, the Director of District Health Administration (Dr. Margaret Barnard) was empowered to delay any technical instruction with which she disagreed for a period of twenty-four hours. During this time she and the bureau director concerned were to work out their differences. Finally, field personnel who took exception to the orders of a district health officer were nevertheless to obey such orders, challenging them by writing to the appropriate bureau chief and submitting a copy to the district health officer.[28] This elaborate order was put out to cover the immediate snowstorm emergency, but was in effect for many years afterward. In general, this order became a dead letter after the snowstorm, and Barnard was unable to assume the authorities granted to her in it. Bureau directors and bureau staff worked around it, undermined it, or openly defied it.[29]

During Mustard's term, construction was begun on the Brownsville Health Center in Brooklyn, and proposals were made for five new health centers. More important, Mustard completely reorganized the department's administrative structure after the Division of Analysis of the Bureau of the Budget had undertaken an extensive study of it. The department's bureaus were grouped into five major divisions: Administration, Environmental Sanitation, Maternal and Child Health, Community Health and Organization, and Preventable Diseases. Each of these broad groups was headed by either a deputy or assistant commissioner. A Bureau of Adult Hygiene was also established at this time.[30]

Another noteworthy accomplishment during Mustard's term was the obtaining of permission to revise the Sanitary Code which, although amended many times, had not been revised in seventy-five years! It would be five years before serious work began on the revision and another five years before it was accomplished.[31]

DECLINE (1950 TO 1953)

It appears that when Mustard resigned in 1949, O'Dwyer, embarrassed by his appointments of Bernecker and Weinstein, was determined to pick a respected health professional to succeed him. On January 1, 1950, he swore in Dr. John F. Mahoney, who had just retired after twenty-one years as director of the United States Public Health Service Venereal Disease Laboratory on Staten Island. In 1943, Mahoney had discovered that penicillin cured syphilis. This was a major medical discovery, and because of it Mahoney enjoyed well-deserved esteem. O'Dwyer, a layman, had no way of knowing that Mahoney's excellence in the laboratory could not be translated into public health administration. For his part, Mahoney was not very keen about accepting the position. In effect, the health commissionership was his retirement job. He did not have great administrative talents, was unable to effectively deal with conflicts within the department, and had no stomach for advocating increased funding to improve and expand the department in order to keep it abreast of the times. He was, however, a pleasant man, a sincere professional of high integrity, and a superb laboratory scientist. But these talents were ill-suited to the health commissionership, and under him the department consequently went into decline.

Mahoney delegated administrative responsibilities to Dr. Samuel Frant, who became his deputy, and to the bureau chiefs. Frant had previously been the Director of the Bureau of Preventable Diseases. In fairness to Mahoney, it should be noted that by the time he took office the department was feeling the cumulative effects of ten years of low salaries, inadequate budgets, and the resultant excessive staff turnover.[32] But Mahoney did not have the talent to turn this situation around.

After O'Dwyer resigned in 1950 and became ambassador to Mexico, he was succeeded by Vincent R. Impelliteri, who won the mayoralty in a special election after he had split with the regular Democrats.[33] Impelliteri was not a dynamic mayor; he simply let the city run on its own steam. No changes were made at the Department of Health, and it, too, marked time.

The department's decline did not go unnoticed. In 1951, the Committee on Public Health of the New York Academy of Medicine sharply criticized Mahoney and the department, noting the latter's obsolete practices, inadequate budgetary control, and poor salaries. It observed that the Bureau of the Budget and the Board of Estimate made decisions without even consulting Mahoney.[34] The watchdog controls of these two groups had been instituted by La Guardia as a means of preventing waste and graft. But as all New York City Health Commissioners have come to learn since, budget examiners intent on achieving fiscal goals and ignorant of public health objectives will make decisions, if allowed, which are frequently not in the best interests of public health. Commissioners must educate budget examiners during the budget formulation process and must fight hard and convincingly for increased allocations and against reductions. In the final analysis, the failure of a commissioner to do so results in the removal of a crucial variable in the budgetary process.

In 1951, the City Council voted $101,700 for an administrative study of the department. Barrington Associates, Inc., a management firm, was asked to evaluate administrative procedures, and the American Public Health Association to conduct a professional assessment of the department.[35] Barrington Associates concluded that the decentralization effort had not succeeded, and recommended that a high degree of decentralization be implemented. Their plan called for giving the district health officer complete control of all activities in his district. The American Public Health Association succinctly stated the status quo in the opening statement of its report: "The Department of Health of New York City was once an outstanding leader in municipal affairs. . . It was one of the best health departments in the country. It no longer is."[36]

In retrospect, Mahoney was simply ill-suited for the commissionership, and the inevitable happened. The department declined. Making this possible was the presence of a mayor like Impelliteri, also content to coast along. O'Dwyer's instincts were well-placed when he picked Mahoney. He was looking for a top public health figure. And although he got that, what he didn't get was a first-rate administrator who could keep the department's machinery up-to-date and effectively deal with the city's larger bureaucratic and political realities.

REVIVAL (1954 TO 1966)

In November 1953, Robert F. Wagner was elected mayor, and he appointed Dr. Leona Baumgartner as Commissioner of Health. She had resigned from her position as Assistant Commissioner for Maternal and Child Health in the department the previous April to become executive director of the New York Foundation. Prior to that, she had spent sixteen years in the department, where she had achieved great success in maternal and child health programs despite budget reductions and cyclical administrative inertia. In no small way, these successes were the result of her own personal qualities, which when brought to bear upon the leadership of the department resulted in its rebirth. Baumgartner combined determination with charm, assertion with warmth, was a splendid administrator, and possessed the ability to make sound judgments. In sum, she was a strong commissioner. Of note is the fact that she was also the department's first female commissioner.

Wagner adopted a policy of noninterference in departmental affairs, a policy he maintained throughout his twelve years as mayor. This policy was abandoned by his successor, Mayor Lindsay, but was resumed afterwards by Mayor Beame in 1974. Both Wagner and Beame left the running of the department to the professionals.

Baumgartner set out to update the department's activities, broaden its scope, and infuse new life into functions that had become dormant. In all of this, she was eminently successful. She appointed Dr. Roscoe P. Kandle as First Deputy Commissioner. He had previously been the Field Director of the American Public Health Association and one of the authors of the report on the department to the Mayor's Committee on Management Survey that had been prepared two years earlier.[37]

Early on, Baumgartner addressed the long-standing controversy between districts and bureaus. She adopted a new policy, which placed the emphasis at the borough level. Both she and Kandle were of the opinion that a neighborhood pattern of health administration was no longer applicable in New York City. This conviction was soundly based on the perception of changed demography, disease patterns, and the unsuitability of the districts as service areas.[38] The Office of District Health Administration became the Office of District Services, with a director reporting to the First Deputy Commissioner. Five borough directors reported to the director of this new office and supervised the district health officers.

Baumgartner, according to Duffy, had an unerring ability to capitalize on dramatic issues and a flair for public relations.[39] These attributes proved to be of great value during field trials for Salk polio vaccine in New York City in 1955, during which 270,000 first- and second-grade children received innoculations.[40] She forged ahead in numerous areas, including both communicable and chronic diseases, program planning and development, and many others. By 1955, she had obtained $100,000 in state and city funds and $60,000 from the Rockefeller Brothers Fund and the W.K. Kellogg Foundation for a three and a half year study of major revisions of the Sanitary Code. On March 23, 1959, the new code, now called the Health Code, was approved by the Board of Health.[41]

She pushed forward with a number of new programs, such as the Diet and Coronary Heart Disease Study Project in 1956, which used the department's Prudent Diet in studying the relationship between nutrition and heart disease. Other programs included glaucoma and diabetes screening and demonstration projects to test health care delivery models.[42]

In September 1958, Mayor Wagner announced the formation of the Health Research Council. Composed of forty-two eminent scientists in the city, the purpose of the Council was to conduct research into the problems of the aged, childbirth and infant care, mental illness, accidents, heart disease, chronic pulmonary disorders, patient care, environmental hazards, and drug addiction.[43] Wagner allocated $600,000 in municipal funds to the new Council and expressed the hope that within four to five years it would be possible to allocate a dollar for every man, woman, and child in the city, or eight million dollars. The Council awarded grants to scientists working in hospitals, medical schools, universities, research institutions, and city departments. It established career scientist awards in an attempt to keep able young researchers in the health field.[44]

On September 22, 1962, President John F. Kennedy announced the appointment of Dr. Baumgartner as assistant administrator for human resources and social development in the U.S. Agency for International Development.[45] Baumgartner had served as Commissioner of Health for the eight years that had witnessed not only major administrative changes, but also strong movement into new frontiers of public health. She had introduced new services and instituted fresh approaches to solving old problems. But, in addition, she created an exciting atmosphere within the department and raised morale to a very high level. Her commissionership was still remembered in the late 1970s by department personnel as a golden period.

Upon her resignation Wagner appointed Dr. George James as Commissioner of Health. James had served as a deputy commissioner under Baumgartner since 1956 and as First Deputy Commissioner since 1959. Like Baumgartner, he possessed enormous energy and a high level of social consciousness. He was both sincere and insightful and did not hesitate to make a frontal assault on a wide assortment of problems. James had previously served for ten years in the New York State Department of Health and, prior to coming to work under Dr. Baumgartner, for one year as Commissioner of Health of Akron, Ohio.

During his time as Baumgartner's deputy, James had focused many of his efforts on the problems of health care organization and delivery. He continued to do so as Commissioner of Health, while carrying on with many of the directions set out by Baumgartner. He opened eight prenatal satellite clinics in districts with high infant mortality rates, and in 1965 assumed direction of medical services for the Department of Corrections. During his tenure, two pilot schemes in health care delivery were begun, the Westchester-Pelham Bay Mental Health Care Project and the Montefiore Prenatal and Infant Care Project. The former was designed to give ambulatory mental health care to patients who would otherwise have been hospitalized. The latter was aimed at determining if nurses could substitute for physicians in providing maternal and child health care.[46] It was during James's administration that the long battle to fluoridate water was finally won, with the help of Mary (Mrs. Albert D.) Lasker, a dedicated New York City philanthropist with a deep concern for health problems. Dr. Howard Rusk, a prominent American physician and Director of the Institute of Rehabilitation Medicine at New York University, was also of enormous assistance to Dr. James in the fluoridation struggle begun during Baumgartner's commissionership.[47]

In June 1965, James announced that he would resign on November 1 in order to accept the position of dean of the newly established Mount Sinai School of Medicine. He served as commissioner for four years, moving the department forward into the newer and pressing problem areas of public health. His departure coincided with the end of the Wagner mayorality and the beginning of John Lindsay's (see Chapter 1). It also heralded the end of an era, for ahead lay troubled social times, turbulent administrative changes, and an erosion of the department's independence and functions.

SUPERAGENCY (1966 TO 1969)

John Lindsay was elected mayor on the Republican ticket with Liberal Party support (see Chapter 1). He was a reform mayor who assumed office at a time when reform was the dominant national mood. A number of President Johnson's Great Society programs were underway, and Medicaid and Medicare, which had both been legislated into existence in 1965, were in the early stages of enactment. Growing demands for a broadening variety of health services, the lowering of financial barriers to medical care, and the development of an array of organizational delivery models introduced new and complex problems with which health administrators had to deal. To their credit, Lindsay and his team were on the cutting edge of this new frontier and were concerned that existing administrative structures could not rise to the new occasion.

One of their first thoughts was, in fact, a very old one that had been tried and abandoned earlier in the century, namely the merger of the Department of Health and Department of Hospitals into one agency. Such a proposal has always provided fertile ground for heated dispute.[48] It was argued that this organizational union would result in functional coordination and elimination of wasteful duplication. But this new structure could not be developed because of a variety of legal and bureaucratic obstacles that would have required years to overcome. Lindsay and his staff then moved in the direction of setting up a superagency to supervise and coordinate the activities of departments in the health field, which included Health, Hospitals, Mental Health, and the Chief Medical Examiners Office.

After James's departure, his First Deputy Commissioner, Dr. John Philp, became Acting Commissioner until December 1965. Philp left the department and was replaced as Acting Commissioner by Dr. Arthur Bushel, one of James's deputies.[49] Bushel was a highly respected public health official, but because he was a dentist and not a medical doctor he did not meet the City Charter requirements for the position of Commissioner of Health.

Meanwhile, a search committee was established for the position of Health Services Administrator. It included a number of eminent health experts, among them Dr. Ernest Stebbins, a former Commissioner of Health of New York City and Dean of the School of Public Health at Johns Hopkins University. The committee recommended Dr. Howard Brown, at the time director of the Ambulatory Care Unit of the Gouverneur Hospital on Manhattan's Lower East Side. Brown had established a model neighborhood health center program that received national attention. Because of the success of this program, in 1964 he was appointed chief medical advisor to the office of Economic Opportunity in Washington, D.C. He set up similar neighborhood health care centers in several cities around the country.[50] Brown was widely respected for his imagination and innovative spirit, qualities the city's health care system needed at this juncture.

Shortly before Brown was appointed on June 1, 1966, Robert Price, Lindsay's former campaign director and now Deputy Mayor, realized that there was no line on which to hire him. It was then that Brown was hired on the Commissioner of Health's vacant line.[51] Because Brown did not have a master's degree in public health or an equivalent degree, he did not meet the City Charter requirements for the Commissioner position. Nonetheless, he occupied it for eight months, until February 16, 1967, when a successor was found.

Obviously, these early administrative maneuvers of the Lindsay team sent very negative signals to the Department of Health's professionals. For, during the first eight-month period of the new administration they were effectively without a full-time commissioner, while a superagency was being conceived of under whose aegis they had a different, if not uncertain, future.

The Health Services Administration was established on June 1, 1966, the day Brown assumed office through the mayor's Executive Order No. 12. A year later, the agency was made statutory under Local Law 127 and ceased to be part of the mayor's office.[52]

In February 1967, eight months after Brown had assumed both the position of Health Services Administrator and that of Commissioner of Health, Lindsay appointed Dr. Edward O'Rourke as Commissioner of Health. O'Rourke had previously served as Commissioner of Health of Cambridge, Massachusetts, from 1951 through 1954, had been a career officer in the United States Public Health Service, and had worked for the United States Agency for International Development. In addition, he had an M.P.H. degree in epidemiology from the Harvard School of Public Health.

Brown was in the unenviable position of trying to exert control over independent department heads. Joseph Terenzio, later president of the United Hospital Fund, was then Commissioner of Hospitals, Dr. Milton Helpern was the city's world renowned Chief Medical Examiner, and Dr. O'Rourke was head of the Department of Health.

In 1966, Lindsay appointed the Commission on the Delivery of Personal Health Services (Piel Commission) and charged it "to make a thorough inquiry into the institutional, administrative and fiscal aspects of the system through which public funds deliver personal health services to one-third of the people of New York City." The following year the Piel Commission recommended the consolidation of the city's health agencies into a single Health Services Administration, and the creation of a politically and financially independent quasi-public benefit corporation to administer the city's public hospitals. On May 26, 1969, the New York State Legislature enacted the New York City Health and Hospitals Corporation Act. This piece of legislation, effective July 1, 1970, created a public benefit corporation to administer the city's public hospitals. It received a great deal of national attention because it represented an important experiment in the organization, administration, and financial management of a large public hospital system.[53]

It is beyond the scope of this presentation to discuss the structure of the Health and Hospitals Corporation (HHC). But it is important to note that the Commissioner of Health was a member of the board, and the Health Services Administrator its chairman. The board's first chairman was Gordon Chase, Lindsay's Health Services Administrator from 1970 through 1973. He was followed by Dr. Lowell Bellin in 1974, whom Mayor Beame appointed both Health Services Administrator and Commissioner of Health. In 1977, this writer was appointed by Beame to succeed Bellin in this triple role. Of significance is the fact that from 1970 on the attention of health commissioners was to some degree diverted to hospital matters because they were members of the HHC board. This responsibility for hospital affairs became even greater for Bellin and this writer, who in addition to being members of the board, also chaired it.

As discussed in Chapter 1, the later 1960s witnessed an enormous expansion of both federal and local spending to deal with the country's burgeoning social problems. The larger environment, in which corrective programs were launched, was characterized by social upheaval, protest, community activism, and demands not only for improved health services, but also for community control of them. Federal initiatives such as Medicaid, Medicare, the Model Cities Program, and the Comprehensive Health Planning Agency placed new deamnds on the Department of Health, demands for which there were no precedents. True, citizens and politicians were concerned about tuberculosis control and nutrition, but few knew of anyone with tuberculosis and malnutrition certainly was rare. But people were concerned about access to health care and its escalating costs, poverty, crime, unemplyoment, and social justice. By the late 1960s, the burning public health issues of a few years before appeared to many as both relatively simple and out-of-date. Understandably, those who were on the firing line during that earlier time would no doubt argue this point. What is not arguable, however, is the inception around 1968 of a tumultuous period of social upheaval, a time of deamnds for change and a rejection of old values and institutions, not without effect on the Department of Health. In the rush to quell this social revolt, galvanized in no small way by the anti-Viet Nam War movement, government came in with expeditious solutions not always easily grafted onto its existing traditional infrastructures. It was far easier to create new agencies to deal with these problems, agencies that were not hampered by legacies of bureaucratic red tape, coasting senior staff, and a reluctance to change.

Many rightly assumed that these new functions could not be integrated into the substance of unwilling health bureaucracies. In no small way, this led to a national rejection of the long-held concept that a health department should have a basic responsibility for everything related to health.[54] If health departments were increasingly left with residual functions not assignable elsewhere, it was often because of their defaulting on the newer challenges. Eventually, even routine functions were carried away, diffused into departments of social services, human services, health systems management, addiction services agencies, and environmental protection agencies. The New York City Department of Health was no exception. Many of its professional staff had come into the department during the Great Depression and were only a few years from retirement. It was easier to coast into that horizon than to wrestle with a host of problems that had exploded from a smoldering state with the upheaval of the late 1960s. Such staff rationalized their decisions not to tackle issues like drug addiction on the grounds that they were not "traditional" public health functions. This, of course, was a surrogate excuse, but one frequently invoked. More and more, the so called "traditional" functions became less important and less relevant as society's focus shifted to the health problems that health departments had left for others to solve.

The growing complexity of health care and the need to bring the varied skills of economists, managers, and planners to bear upon current health problems resulted in an erosion of the primacy of the public health physician. Good nonphysician managers and planners performed as well, and even better at times, than did physicians, destroying the mystique that only physicians could do these jobs. Additionally, young nonphysician managers brought to their tasks a daring and dynamism often lacking in older public health physicians.

In early 1968, Dr. Howard Brown resigned as Health Services Administrator. As he recounts it in his autobiography, *Familiar Faces, Hidden Lives*, he was in St. Vincent's Hospital with acute hepatitis when his brother-in-law, a reporter for *The New York Times*, informed him that an investigative reporter might be planning to expose homosexuals in Mayor Lindsay's administration.[55] Brown, who publicly announced his homosexuality in October 1973, was fearful of exposure and consequently resigned.[56] Lindsay appointed Dr. Bernard Bucove, a highly respected public health physician, to succeed him as Health Services Administrator. O'Rourke continued as Commissioner of Health for another year an a half until June, 1969, when he was replaced by Dr. Mary C. McLaughlin, his deputy. Dr. McLaughlin had been with the department for almost twenty years and had served in a variety of positions, including those of health officer, district health officer, Borough Director of Queens, Assistant Commissioner, and Deputy Commissioner. She brought to the health commissionership an extensive knowledge of the department and of the city's community health problems, in addition to managerial and administrative talents developed from years of experience.

Mayor Lindsay successfully ran again in 1969. Much of his attention during the following three years was focused on what turned out to be an unsuccessful presidential bid. In the health field, however, major changes were about to take place. Under Brown and Bucove, the Health Services Administration had virtually no staff and no control over the budgeting and personnel functions of its operating agencies.[57] Lindsay had not been pleased by the performance of the agency and, according to Morris, thought that it needed management at the top more than medical expertise.[58] It can be argued of course, that Lindsay, with an eye toward the presidency, was eager to ride public health issues to political success. In order to do so he had to have leadership at the Health Services Administration that was loyal, responsive to his political needs, and capable of producing results that could be translated into positive media coverage. Physician administrators, as Lindsay knew, were a mixed blessing, combining expertise with allegiance to professional standards and goals. Their loyalty could not be counted on, especially if it came into conflict with professional standards.[59]

In 1970, Lindsay started his second term by replacing Dr. Bernard Bucove as Health Services Administrator with a nonphysician, Gordon Chase. Bucove then became Director of the School of Hygiene at the University of Toronto. Chase was a highly respected manager who had gained a reputation by cleaning up serious financial disorders at the city's Human Resources Administration.[60] He was also a loyal Lindsay supporter. Over the next four years he radically transformed the Health Services Administration into a large functioning superagency with a broad spectrum of direct program responsibilities.

Chapter 4

THE HEALTH SERVICES ADMINISTRATION

The structure and functions of the Health Service Administration (HSA) during the four-year period 1970 to 1973 were overwhelmingly imprinted with Gordon Chase's style of management. Morris has accurately characterized Chase as a devotee of project management. His style was to break a program down into discrete projects, which were then brought to completion by project managers who operated outside the normal bureaucratic chain of command.[1] Project managers reported directly to Chase and, in so doing, often bypassed the professionals responsible for programs. This enabled Chase to achieve high visibility and claim rapid success by overcoming perceived bureaucratic obstacles.[2] Chase consistently excluded the Department of Health's professionals from major policy formulation and, in time, took over the running of many of the department's activities through program analysts hired by the HSA. As Bellin has pointed out, the formal table of organization still showed the program analysts as having the role of supportive staff to health professionals. But, in point of fact, the antithesis was true.[3]

THE POLITICAL ENVIRONMENT

What transpired within the HSA and the Department of Health during Chase's four-year tenure was not merely the result of a commitment to a specific management style. It was also the result of loyalty to a reform mayor actively seeking the Democratic party's nomination for President. In the final analysis, Chase's style, resulting as it did in high public visibility for claimed successes, served this political end quite well. This does not, of course, represent a sweeping indictment of Chase's administration. But it does cast some doubt on his claimed successes, and raises the obvious question about his motives for adopting a project management style.

Leveson and Weiss state that there were a number of constraints on the abilities of superagency administrators to bring about change. They list as the first and perhaps most important the varied and powerful news media.[4] They point out that Lindsay's administration was probably more concerned than most about its local and national press coverage because Lindsay was either contemplating or was actually running for President.[5] The pervasive news coverage of local issues gave administrators "a strong incentive to avoid or hide situations which might turn up in the press as problems."[6] They claim that this was a powerful incentive to avoid correcting mistakes because the media was prone to focus on the problem rather than on the corrective action.[7]

They also relate that Chase was constrained in his actions regarding the HHC. This was because he was not a line administrator in the HHC, merely its board chairman. Additionally, Lindsay's reputation was on the line since he was clearly associated with both the establishment of the HHC and the hiring of its president.[8] Negative press stories about the HHC reflected badly on the mayor. Under normal circumstances, mayors have sustained their share of criticism for the failures of the HHC. But a presidential candidate such as Lindsay perceived that he could ill-afford to sustain any. Thus, as Leveson and Weiss state, confrontations between HHC and HSA were avoided over a host of issues in order to project an image of the HHC as an effective and successful accomplishment in institutional change.[9] In effect, loyalty and responsiveness to the mayor's political goals often took precedence over loyalty to professional goals.

Sayre and Kaufman have cogently stated that elected officials have learned to mistrust the loyalty of appointed professionals because of the latter's allegiance to the standards of a peer group outside the immediate hierarchical governmental network.[10] Bellin convincingly argues that the most effective government is one in which healthy tension persists between the elected official and the appointed professional. He goes on to say that when this tension has dissipated, one can assume that either one, or the other, or both are playing their roles poorly.[11] In sum, this is what occurred in the HSA during Lindsay's second term.

STRUCTURE

The HSA eventually became the superagency governing four separate city departments and the semi-autonomous HHC. These departments included Health, Mental Health, the Addiction Services Agency, and the Office of the Chief Medical Examiner. Additionally, the HSA administrator became chairman of both the board and the executive committee of the Comprehensive Health Planning Agency (CHPA). As Leveson and Weiss explain, the CHPA was engaged in organizing local community planning bodies and in maintaining its own viability during most of Chase's tenure. The organization did not engage in effective planning or lobbying during his administration, but it did take up a significant amount of his time.[12]

The internal structure of the HSA consisted of four major divisions, Health Research, Management Services, Program Analysis, Planning and Budgeting, and Legal.[13] In addition, a Public Information and Health Education Office reported directly to the administrator. This structure was appropriate to the agency's mandate, which was data collection and analysis, and coordination and rationalization of overall health policy. Gradually, however, the HSA staff encroached on the daily operations of the delegated agencies, especially those of the Department of Health. This had several effects, among which were a denigration of the position of the Commissioner of Health and a sense of role ambiguity among middle and lower ranks in the delegated departments.[14]

PERSONNEL

A detailed profile of the personnel hired to work for the HSA is given by Leveson and Weiss, both of whom held high positions within the agency. They state that staff members were generally well-educated and highly motivated, but that with few exceptions they did not have substantial prior experience or education in the health services area.[15] It is useful to pause for a while and examine this general profile. The characterization "well-educated" refers to individuals who often had only undergraduate baccalaureate degrees in a variety of areas including English, History, Political Science, and Mathematics. Few would argue that they were not well-educated, but many would question the suitability of the education to the responsibilities eventually given to them.

Leveson and Weiss say that there were several reasons for few people with health backgrounds on the HSA analysis staff. They cite a salary structure that would not support the hiring of many first-rate experienced persons with health backgrounds.[16] This contention, however, does not hold up under close scrutiny; four years later it was possible to hire such persons on the same salary scales. They also claim that physicians were too expensive and typically lacked the training and inclination to do policy analysis.[17] True, there were physicians who did not have such skills and others whom the HSA could not recruit because of low salary scales. But, there were physicians who were both skilled and experienced in policy analysis already on the staff of the Department of Health or willing to join the HSA ranks from the outside. Yet their talents were never recruited. Leveson and Weiss claim that the young professionals with health backgrounds in the labor market, such as those with master's degrees in public health, tended not to have the kind of training that would prepare them well for policy analysis positions.[18]

In a related vein, they add that, at the time, many schools of public health did not attract the best quality students.[19] This is a sweeping indictment of both the schools of public health and their graduates, and one that cannot be sustained by hard facts. Leveson and Weiss go on to say that when they were presented with a choice between less capable persons with health backgrounds and more analytic persons without health experience or training, they often chose the latter.[20] They subscribe to the opinion that generalized health knowledge is often superfluous when dealing with highly particularized problems in a rapidly changing context. Few health professionals would agree with this argument.

When Dr. Lowell Bellin became Health Services Administrator in 1974, he found that among a total of twenty-four HSA program analysts not a single one possessed the Master of Public Health degree or an equivalent Master of Business Administration or Master of Public Administration degree.[21] In effect, as Bellin states, committed amateurism and spontaneity had supplanted relevant education and experience in health affairs.[22] He goes on to say that the staffing policy of the superagency had effectively isolated policy decisions from the influence of health professionals.[23]

In looking back over the expanse of the decade since the HSA was formed, it is easier to discern that the staff was a heterogeneous mix. It included qualified analysts and economists with both training and experience, young inexperienced and untrained enthusiasts of Lindsay's reform policies, and preelection loyalists of the mayor in need of jobs. Health professionals were a minority on the HSA staff, and those within the Department of Health were effectively cut off from policy formulation processes. It is reasonable to ask why Chase chose not to utilize the talents of professionals already in the Department of Health. Granted, there were some who had retreated from the burgeoning, newer public health problems. But there were also others who had not. And certainly, contrary to what Leveson and Weiss claim, there were qualified, and experienced health professionals who could have been recruited. The answer to this question is rather clear when one realizes that what actually took place was a substantial politicization of public health structure and functions. This was really a very old maneuver, but unlike previous efforts, it was accomplished with a new twist, namely managerialism. Professionals have always been a major obstacle to politicization and notoriously uncooperative with mayors and administrators who have tried to foist it on them. It was accomplished in the HSA during the years 1970 to 1973 by the exclusion of professionals and the use of managerial rhetoric and techniques as a mantle of respectability. This is not to say that these managerial techniques did not bring about some excellent results in specific program areas. But in many other areas they and the politicization process with which they were intimately intertwined eventually caused a deprofessionalization of public health in the city.

THE EFFECT OF THE HSA ON THE DEPARTMENT OF HEALTH

Although program analysts were originally recruited to analyze programs and provide information to be used in the decision-making process, they eventually came to formulate many of the Department of Health's policies. In addition, a number assumed direct responsibility for administering programs or positions of them, divorced from the department's professionals. Chase wanted fast results, which could be readily translated into high visibility assets for the mayor. The involvement of professionals served as an impediment to this goal. And so there was a conscious effort to exclude them as much as possible.

When Bellin became Acting Health Services Administrator and Commissioner of Health in January 1974, he found that the department had been deprofessionalized. Some health professionals had resigned because of policies that were incompatible with normative standards of public health administration.[24] Some had shamefully compromised their standards, either to curry favor or in an effort to hold on to their jobs.[25] Others had used imaginative guile to preserve the professional integrity of the programs entrusted to them. And still others had used a mixture of defiance and bluff to head off the incursions of aggressive program analysts.[26]

Dr. Mary C. McLaughlin, who had become Commissioner of Health in July 1969, served in the position until January 1972, when Chase succeeded in replacing her. McLaughlin had mounted a sustained and effective opposition to the HSA's deprofessionalization and politicization efforts for almost two years. She also made a valiant effort to preserve professional standards and recruit and retain professional staff. To Chase she was a major professional obstacle, enhanced by her years of experience in the department and the loyalty and support of the professional staff. She was replaced by Dr. Joseph A. Cimino, McLaughlin's First Deputy Commissioner, for a few weeks. Cimino had extensive training and experience in occupational and industrial health, including a Master of Public Health degree from the Harvard School of Public Health. To a certain degree, he shared Chase's philosophy about project management, and during his tenure, program analysts assumed greater control of the department's professional activities.

During McLaughlin's tenure, Chase had diverted Department of Health funds to support the costs of HSA programs and staff. This continued under Cimino.[27] The authority of the Commissioner of Health and the bureau chiefs diminished due to loss of staff, restrictions on hiring, and the inability to begin new projects.[28] Bureaus that had once directed services were bypassed; for example, treatment services were introduced into child health stations with no involvement of the Bureau of Child Health.[29]

Program analysts produced an enormous number of reports concerning departmental programs. Some of these, such as those dealing with prison health, were of high quality and were extremely useful in bringing about necessary administrative reforms.[30] Others, however, were of inferior quality, and some were politically motivated. For example, HSA undertook a hypertension screening program without any prior study because it appeared obvious on the basis of existing information that hypertension screening was a politically and programmatically appropriate course of action.[31] Weiss relates that in numerous instances the HSA program staff undertook studies that led to or facilitated programmatic changes despite the lack of any real knowledge of the link between changes in the program design and changes in performance indicators.[32] He also states that in some instances prior political commitments to a particular program design necessitated that the program evaluation be ignored.[33] This combination of political expediency and amateurism often resulted in poor program design and has cast suspicion, in an historical sense, over all of the HSA programs, even those that were appropriately designed to meet current public health needs.

One of the most important changes in the Department of Health during Cimino's term was the complete reorganization of district health services. As has been pointed out several times in previous chapters, other commissioners had attempted to deal with this thorny problem. At the heart of it lay the inherent conflicts between strong bureau directors and district health officers. However, by 1972, when the new plan was implemented, the powers of the bureau directors had been greatly reduced and they themselves had been effectively isolated from many main stream policy decisions. Thus, the long standing problem of bureau director/district health officer conflict was minimal.

In 1971, program analysts from the HSA studied service provision at a district health center and found poorly administered clinics with no single person held accountable for performance.[34] The study recommended that one individual be assigned responsibility for district health center operations and that a reporting system be developed for measuring and evaluating services.[35] The following year Commissioner Cimino and his First Deputy Commissioner, Alan Gibbs, began what became the most significant change in the management of district health services since the 1930s. Gibbs, who was not a physician, was an able administrator widely respected for his managerial talents. Although he reported directly to the Commissioner of Health according to the formal organization chart, he also informally reported directly to the HSA administrators who had chosen him for the position. This line of command gave Chase direct access to the department's enormous district health services network, an access that had been previously blocked by Dr. McLaughlin.

Cimino and Gibbs set out to overcome many of the obstacles to previous attempts at reorganizing district services.[36] Initially, they reviewed all of the programs, policies, and services of the bureaus and met with both the district health officers and the bureau directors in order to prepare them for the administrative changes.[37] In a symbolic gesture, Cimino held general staff meetings at district health centers. At the first of these, which was held at a center in Brooklyn, he announced that "the day of the districts has arrived." The plan for administrative decentralization of personal health services included the transfer of budgetary authority for local services to districts, the establishment of a district cost accounting system, and the appointment of district health managers.[38] After considerable discussion within the department, Cimino issued an executive order requesting that the bureau directors submit a list of functions over which they wished to retain control and the reasons therefor.[39] Eventually, the redefined role of the bureaus in district services was that of standard-setting evaluation. There were some exceptions to this, such as the functions of the Bureau for Handicapped Children.

Most bureau directors resisted these attempts to strip them of operational responsibilities. But Cimino lent his support to the district health officers whenever conflicts arose, much the same as Dr. John Rice had lent his to bureau directors thirty years before. A Health Officers Advisory Committee was formed, through which the district health officers regularly met with both the Commissioner and the bureau directors.[40]

Reorganization also took place in each district. Gibbs recruited district health managers, a new category of health personnel who were assigned to health centers after being approved by the health officer. By July 1973, twenty of the department's twenty-two centers had managers. Overall, these individuals proved to be of very high quality. They were responsible for the operation of all administrative and clinical services in the districts.[41] In principle, they were supervised by the health officer. But the district managers had an official line of communication to Alan Gibbs, the First Deputy Commissioner, who held them directly responsible for district operations.[42] This line bypassed the district health officers and the Deputy Commissioner for District Health Services.

Other aspects of the reorganization of district health services included the institution of a district reporting and accounting system, which provided clinic utilization and unit cost data on a decentralized basis by districts.[43] Additionally, program budgeting was introduced, and the purchasing of supplies was decentralized. As Mustalish, Eidsvold, and Novick have reported, by the fall of 1973 health officers and managers had authority and accountability for operations, personnel actions, purchasing, budgeting, and program administration.[44] The role of the bureaus was largely advisory, consultative, and evaluative.[45] But new problems replaced the old ones. Health officer/health manager conflicts filled the void left by the old frictions between health officers and bureau directors. Also, the First Deputy's span of control over sixteen health officers and twenty-two managers was too wide to permit effective administration. In an attempt to remedy this latter situation, Cimino and Gibbs established six regions, each headed by a regional health director who was a former district health officer. Each of these regional health directors replaced the borough health directors and had two district health officers and four managers reporting to them. The regional health directors in turn reported to the First Deputy Commissioner. The managers were given operational responsibility for district activities, while the health officers served as staff to the regional directors on program planning and evaluation.[46] These administrative changes, which went into effect in November 1973, clearly shifted ultimate responsibility and authority from health officers to managers, and placed health officers in staff positions which isolated them from daily operational decisions. And although the six regional health directors reported directly to the First Deputy Commissioner, so did all the health managers. Thus, by 1973 both categories of professionals—bureau directors and health officers—were neatly quarantined from a broad scope of operations and policy decisions. This left a clear field for the HSA staff to utilize the district infrastructure for implementing and modifying programs with not just professional goals in mind.

At the central office, HSA control of bureau functions was not only achieved by analysts seizing portions of programs or entire programs, but also by the insertion of HSA loyal nonprofessionals into bureau director, assistant commissioner, and deputy commissioner positions. By mid-1973 Chase had consolidated his control of most areas of the department, except for those in which formidable resistance had been mounted by professionals or those in which activities could not easily be ridden to political success.

ACCOMPLISHMENTS OF THE HSA

It is not easy to assess Chase's administration, for like Royal Copeland, a Commissioner of Health of fifty years before, he was an outspoken fighter for public health and welfare.[47] To his credit, he organized the city's methadone maintenance treatment program, created a Bureau of Lead Poison Control within the Department of Health, and implemented much needed accounting and reporting systems in district services. He reorganized and automated the vital statistics division of the department, mounted programs against sickle cell anemia, hypertension, and alcoholism, and revamped the rat control program. Under his aegis the new abortion program was developed, and HSA took over a scandalously deteriorated prison health program.[48] Like Royal Copeland, he had a keen sense of public relations and managed to get maximum media coverage in the service of Mayor Lindsay's political ambitions. But in the process he politicized the Department of Health and presided over its deprofessionalization. This is not to imply that all of Chase's undertakings were politically motivated. Far from it. Many were spawned from his own strong commitment to public welfare and reform and from his desire to apply management techniques to problems that had long proven intractable to all else.

But enthusiasm is no replacement for experience and training, nor management a substitute for professionalism. Lacking in Chase's administration was a healthy balance of managerialism and professionalism and a strong concern for professional standards. Duffy, in assessing Royal Copeland's record, says that a good health commissioner needs to be aware of, and sensitive to, political relations, but that his goals should be professionally oriented.[49] Like Copeland, Chase had an excessive concern for political goals which, despite some of the splendid managerial techniques he used to promote public health, were the driving engine of his administration. As

Copeland had done a half century before, he tried to ride public health and welfare issues to political success; in the process, he deprofessionalized the Department of Health and opened the way for political interference.[50]

Chapter 5

REPROFESSIONALIZATION, THE FISCAL CRISIS, AND THE KOCH ADMINISTRATION

In the fall of 1973, Abraham D. Beame, for two terms the city's comptroller, was elected mayor on the Democratic ticket. John V. Lindsay, who had withdrawn from the Democratic primary race for the Presidency the preceding year, did not run for the mayoralty. Beame's campaign platform included not only a commitment to abolish the costly and duplicative superagencies, but also to reprofessionalize the Department of Health. Like Mayor Wagner, Beame subscribed to a public policy of placing public health in the hands of professionals. And like Wagner, he did not interfere in the affairs of the Department of Health.

In order to find a new health commissioner, Beame established a large search committee whose members included Dr. Howard Rusk and Dr. Mary McLaughlin, then Commissioner of Health of the Suffolk County Health Services Department. They recommended that he appoint Dr. Lowell E. Bellin, then Professor of Public Health and Chairman of the Division of Health Administration at Columbia University's School of Public Health. Bellin, who assumed the dual positions of Commissioner of Health and Acting Health Services Administrator on January 7, 1974, was a distinguished public health figure with a national reputation. A trained internist and cardiologist, he had obtained a masters degree in public health from the Harvard School of Public Health in 1964, and had served as Commissioner of Health of Springfield, Massachusetts, from 1962 through 1966. He then became the Associate Medical Director of the Health Insurance Plan of Greater New York, and in 1967 was appointed Executive Director of the New York City Medicaid Program within the Department of Health. There he established a national reputation for standard setting and quality assurance, and shaped a model program that was subsequently copied in other areas of the country. Then, in 1969 Dr. Mary McLaughlin appointed him First Deputy Commissioner, a position in which he served until early 1972 when he left to join the faculty at Columbia.

Mayor Beame's charge to Bellin was to reprofessionalize and upgrade the Department of Health. This Bellin proceeded to do with unusual speed and efficiency. Beame also requested that he dismantle the Health Services Agency (HSA). Most of the top executives of the HSA had exited in the waning days of the Lindsay administration. Gordon Chase left in the fall of 1973, being succeeded by his First Deputy Administrator, Gerald Frug, an attorney. Bellin's principal administrative challenges were to reorganize the Department of Health, dismantle the HSA structure and, in his capacity as Chairman of the Board of the Health and Hospitals Corporation (HHC), deal with steadily deteriorating conditions in this nineteen-institution organization.

In the last year of Chase's administration, numerous administrative structural changes were made in the Department of Health at frequent intervals. These resulted in confusing chains of command, in which a given bureau director often reported to more than one assistant commissioner. An ever-expanding number of titles was given to nonprofessional loyalists as reward for even mediocre performance. As Bellin points out, modestly competent achievements produced rapid and easy promotion.[1] Many professionals within the department suspected that the titles were given in an attempt to aggrandize the recipients' résumés. Whatever the reason, the end result was a good deal of administrative chaos.

Bellin had a unique ability to combine professionalism with sound management and, to his credit, he took the pains to evaluate the remaining HSA program analyst and managerial staff. He found some individuals of excellent quality and integrated them into the Department of Health's reorganized structure. As he himself points out, some of these potentially good people had peaked too soon and had become accustomed to dealing directly with the HSA administrator.[2] They found it difficult to report to superiors lower in the chain of command.

REBIRTH OF THE DEPARTMENT OF HEALTH

In his first week in office, Bellin reorganized district health services. He appointed a Deputy Commissioner for District Services and retained the regional structure previously established, but placed health officers in charge of each district with managers reporting to them. Health officers and regional health directors were given expanded roles in monitoring and evaluation functions and in representing the department in area councils of the developing Health Systems Agency. Simultaneously, he restructured the department and began recruiting a large number of well-trained and experienced professionals who came from both within and outside the department.

The rebirth of the department, which took place during 1974, was comparable, according to older departmental staff, to what had occurred when John Rice was commissioner and Leona Baumgartner assumed the commissionership in 1954. What characterized this rebirth was not only administrative reorganization, but also the infusion of professional leadership into the department. And in place of the confusing and chaotic chains of command that existed previously, Bellin established a clear-cut and unambiguous administrative structure. This included five deputy commissioners for Management and Budget, Professional Standards and Review, Health Institutions and Environmental Health Services, District Health Services, and Substance Abuse Services. There were also six associate and assistant commissioners for Medicaid, Biostatistics and Research, Maternal and Child Health, Public Health Nursing, Laboratory Services, and Chronic and Communicable Diseases. Various bureau directors reported to these levels. In addition, Bellin recruited an Executive Medical Director for Prison Health Services and a Director for what would become the unique New York City Employee Counseling Service.

Bellin appointed a trained and experienced physician as First Deputy Commissioner to oversee the daily operations of the department. With the exception of the Deputy Commissioner for Management and Budget, all of the deputy commissioners reported to him. It was Bellin's policy to delegate high levels of responsibility and decision making to his deputies. This, coupled with the excellence of the people he recruited, resulted in imaginative new programs and the efficient operation of the department according to the highest professional standards. It was Bellin's view that the department would have to expand into the area of quality control. During his earlier years with the department, he had launched the Medicaid quality control program of promulgating, monitoring, and enforcing standards of health care delivery. The department later extended these activities to the ambulatory services of 22 voluntary hospitals under the terms of the Ghetto Medicine Program. This program, aimed at subsidizing medical care for the poor, was later extended to 32 voluntary hospitals and the outpatient services of some of the city's municipal hospitals and Health Insurance Plan. He reasonably argued for an expanded health department role in quality control. He stated that "the Health Department must assume responsibility for watching over quality of all types of health care, whether this care is administered under public or even under so called private auspices."[3]

Some have erroneously interpreted this position, which was also shared by Bellin's successor, this writer, as representing a philosophical opposition to providing direct personal services.[4] Because of this alleged position, so the argument goes, coupled with the state health department's assumption of city department functions and the fiscal crisis, the Department of Health was virtually dismantled as a major force in New York's health scene.[5] This interpretation of the Bellin administration's public policy toward personal health services is without any foundation, and is relied upon to provide a simplistic interpretation for the complex array of national and local policies and events that had an impact on the department's personal health services.

Bellin and his staff viewed quality control as an expanding frontier for a department that already had a distinguished record of years of experience in the area. Placing emphasis on quality control was not incompatible with the continuance of needed personal health services. With regard to the latter, however, it had been observed that in a number of health districts there had been a steady decline in the demand for certain of these services. This decline was due to lower disease prevalence; for example, tuberculosis, the development of alternate provider sources and, very important, the removal of financial barriers to medical care because of Medicaid, Medicare, and the Ghetto Medicine Program. People who were once only able to obtain certain services at Department of Health facilities were now able to obtain them from other providers. True, some departmental preventive services were unique, but others, such as certain categories of treatment programs, were not. In addition, there were stronger hopes for national health insurance in the early and mid-1970s. Understandably, Bellin and his staff reasoned that under any program of reasonably extensive national health insurance, demand for free health department services would fall, and it would be fiscally impossible to justify the continuance of such free services for people who could pay for them elsewhere. The rationalizing of these services as the last resort of the poor would no longer be valid.

It is easy to see, then, why Bellin and his staff adopted a policy of expanding in the area of quality control and of maintaining personal health services to meet needs. This policy was, of course, readjusted during the fiscal crisis and afterwards when it became apparent that such expansion would not be possible. This was not only the result of the fiscal crisis, but more important, because of the steady erosion by the New York State Health Department of the city department's regulatory and standard-setting functions. Similarly, as hopes for national health insurance grew dimmer, it was realized that the department would have to maintain significant levels of personal health services for the forseeable future.

DISSOLUTION OF THE HSA

Mayor Beame apointed Bellin as both Commissioner of Health and Acting Health Services Administrator. The latter designation had a threefold purpose: to enable Bellin to supervise activities and programs of the HSA while simultaneously dismantling it, and to fill the position of Chairman of the HHC board. Abolition of the HSA required the approval of the City Council and posed a difficult legal problem with regard to the HHC board. The HHC act of 1969

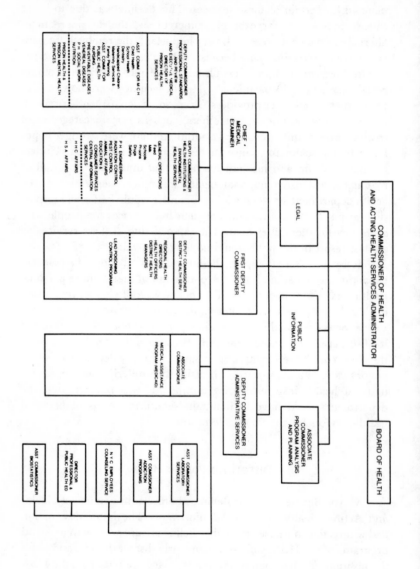

Figure 5-1   Organization Chart for the New York City
Department of Health, 1977

specifically legislated the HSA administrator as chairman. Could there be an HSA administrator without an HSA? This question arose on a number of occasions during 1976 and 1977. The Beame administration was understandably unwilling to push for the introduction of an amendment to the HHC act in the state legislature. To do so would have opened the door for a number of single-issue and single-institution constituencies to push for self-serving amendments which would have had a deleterious impact on a greatly troubled system. And there was always the possibility that some legislators, responding to constituent pressures, would try to amend the act so as to exclude or minimize city control. This was unacceptable to a city administration that was subsidizing the HHC and absorbing its ever-growing annual deficits.

Legal opinion held that the position of HSA administrator could exist without a functioning HSA. This meant that the HHC Act would not have to be amended to provide a new chairman of the board or a process for selecting one.[6] The mayor's stated intent to abolish the HSA, and Bellin's confirmation of this during his first weeks in office, resulted in the desired resignation of the heavy layers of executives and managers of which the agency was primarily composed, and tax-levy savings of close to $ two million.[7]

The HSA was not legally abolished by an act of the City Council until 1977, although it ceased to be a functioning reality six months after Bellin assumed office.[8] Local Law 25, which abolished the HSA, also established two independent departments of Health, Mental Health, Mental Retardation, and Alcoholism Services, and provided for the absorption of the Addiction Services Agency by the Department of Health.[9] The Chief Medical Examiner also reported to the Commissioner of Health. On December 2, 1977, Mayor Beame issued an executive order transferring the powers and duties of the HSA administrator as specified in Chapter 1016 of the 1969 law to the Commissioner of Health.[10]

During Beame's administration, both Bellin and this writer simultaneously served as Commissioner of Health, Acting Health Services Administrator, Chairman of the Board of the HHC, Chairman of the Executive Committee of the Health Systems Agency, and Chairman of the Inter-Agency Health Council. The last named was composed of all city agencies involved in health matters, including the Human Resources Administration.

MAJOR ACCOMPLISHMENTS

In addition to reprofessionalizing the Department of Health and overseeing the enormous task of restructuring the city's public health services, Bellin, as HHC board chairman, had to devote an enormous amount of time and effort to the mounting fiscal, managerial, and medical care quality problems of the city's municipal hospitals. Additionally, he had to actively participate in the formation of the Health Systems Agency and, because of his input, the bylaws were written so that the Commissioner of Health would serve as either chairman of the executive committee or chairman of the board.

During his tenure, the Management by Objective program and the Integrated Financial Management System were gradually introduced into the Department of Health. Bellin introduced Board of Health legislation concerning window guards for the prevention of falls by young children, prevention of the transport of nuclear wastes through the city, and prevention of the burning of high sulfur containing fuels by the local utility company. During most of 1976, the department was involved in the Swine Flu immunization program.[11]

THE FISCAL CRISIS

The spectacular progress of 1974 was halted by the fiscal crisis which began late in the year. During the ensuing 18 months, the city implemented drastic measures to deal with a large budgetary deficit that had developed over so many years. These measures included the establishment of the Emergency Financial Control Board to oversee and monitor the city's financial plans, and the development of the Municipal Assistance Corporation to deal with the city's bonds and notes.

The city's financial deficits had grown steadily for at least two decades. Until 1974 deficit spending had been possible because the city could raise the monies it needed through the sale of short-term notes and longer term bonds. The debts eventually accrued, and added to the ever-growing debts caused by the rising costs of liberal city services, placed the city near bankruptcy. New York City had, until that time, provided a high level of social and medical services, but did not have the tax base to provide these high levels of service. Further complicating the city's financial situation was the high demand generated by a growing indigent population for free services.

In 1975, approximately 938,000 of the city's total population of 7.8 million were indigent, that is, on welfare. Most were recent arrivals from rural southern states and the Caribbean islands. The cost of supporting this population and/or providing them with a wide variety of services was enormous. The complex reasons for the steady inflow of the poor into such large urban centers as New York City are beyond the scope of this discussion. This demographic shift has been occurring on a major scale for the past two decades, accompanied by an exodus of the middle class to the suburbs. For other varied reasons, industry and commerce have also gradually been flowing out of the city to distant or nearby suburbs. The most important net impact of all these shifts is a dwindling of the city's tax base at a time when there is an enormous demand for tax-supported services (see Chapter 1).

THE CITY'S EXPENSE BUDGET

In 1975, the city's total expense budget was $13,084,800,000. Of this $13 billion $2.8 billion were allocated to the Human Resources Administration and $1.2 billion to the Health and Hospitals Corporation, the public municipal hospital system. Thus, 31 percent of the city's operating budget went into human services. Table 5-1 shows the appropriations of the city's 1975 expense budget. Health services include the $1.2 billion allocation for the Health and Hospitals Corporation, $90 million for the Department of Health, and the remainder for the Addiction Services Agency and the Department of Mental Health and Mental Retardation. The Department of Health's budget of $90 million was rather modest when compared with the $1.2 billion for the Health and Hospitals Corporation, the $2.7 billion for education, and the $2.8 billion for human resources. Of this $90 million, only $40 million was tax-levy money, that is, money raised directly by the city through taxes. The remaining $50 million was money received by the department primarily through federal government grants for specific programs.

MUNICIPAL BUDGET RETRENCHMENT

To deal with the fiscal crisis, city, state, and federal officials moved on a number of fronts in 1975 to balance the city's budget by fiscal year 1978. In September 1975 the governor of New York signed

Table 5-1

Appropriations of the 1975 New York City Expense
Budget

	Amount*
Education	$ 2,771.00
Human resources	2,823.30
Health services	1,328.70
Police	908.40
City University	584.90
Charitable institutions	517.30
Environmental protection	391.50
Fire	388.80
Courts	154.30
Municipal services	119.00
Transportation	111.20
Correction	93.20
Housing and Development	81.00
Libraries	54.30
Finance	36.90
Economic development	9.20
All other agencies	183.90
Debt services	1,510.20
Miscellaneous	918.40
TOTAL	$13,084.80

*millions of dollars

a bill creating the Emergency Financial Control Board, which
required, among other things, that the city submit a detailed financial
plan to the board. The plan encompassed the three fiscal years ending
June 30 1976, 1977, and 1978 (the city's fiscal year runs from July 1
to June 30). The expense budget had to be cut by $200 million for
each of these three years.

Budget reductions were difficult for many reasons. Reductions take away jobs, career opportunities, and political and community power bases. Those with vested interests in these areas rarely articulate their opposition to reductions in terms of these losses, but decry the loss of the services that budget reductions will cause. This had great appeal in 1975 to a population accustomed to levels of city services far above those elsewhere in the United States. Thus, the implementation of budget cuts in 1975 took place in a strongly emotion-charged political atmosphere.

The general public was only too willing to believe that the city's fiscal crisis was due to incompetence, graft, corruption, inefficiency, and poor planning. The media and press often lent credence to these simplistic and erroneous notions by recounting isolated tales of bureaucrats coming to work at 9:30 A.M. and leaving at 4:30 P.M., and by depicting pothole fillers as shopping during working hours. The occasional indictment of a public official for misconduct, corruption, or embezzlement supported this view. That many such indictments were dismissed was not generally disclosed by the kind of headlines that announced them. By 1976 these simplistic explanations had poor currency among those who realized the greater social and economic problems at the center of the city's fiscal crisis (see Chapter 1).

Most of the city's operating expense budget cannot, by and large, be controlled. Such costs as public assistance (welfare), Medicaid payments, debt service, and pension contributions are mandated by law. Hence, budget cuts were limited to expenses over which the city does have control. In the 1975 operating budget, only $3.4 billion (26 percent) of the $13 billion total was controllable. And in this area the city's control varied enormously from complete to indirect or weak.

The city's financial plan not only encompassed budget reductions, but also management reforms and a new budgeting system. To achieve these long-term goals, outside experts and consultants were brought in on loan from industry, some to serve gratis at the deputy mayor level. City agencies were eventually integrated into the Management by Objective Program and the Integrated Financial Management System.

To meet the immediate demands of reducing the expense budget, city agencies had to implement a number of changes. These fell into the following broad areas: changes in basic administrative structure to increase efficiency and savings, elimination and reduction of selected programs, reductions in such nonpersonnel costs as equipment and rent, achievement of operational efficiencies, and accelerated attrition of personnel by early retirement.

RETRENCHMENT WITHIN THE DEPARTMENT OF HEALTH

When the fiscal crisis first emerged in November 1974, the city's Office of Management and Budget requested that the Department of Health reduce its work force by 67 employees to save $1.5 million in tax-levy monies. This request was part of the overall reductions levied against all city agencies, not only to produce savings and budget retrenchment, but also to demonstrate the city's determination to balance its budget. This was crucial to the city's bid for state and federal assistance. The credibility of the city's efforts hinged upon rapid budget retrenchment.

This initial request came when the specter of default on bonds and notes was an immediate concern, and when there were doubts that the city could meet its next payroll. Even when it did the latter, some New York banks refused to accept the checks. Numerous employees came to the office of this writer reporting that banks refused to either cash or accept their pay checks for deposit. The need to defuse inordinate panic was urgent, and one method used was the immediate announcement of budget cuts.

It is a staple of every administrative handbook that budget reductions be implemented after careful study of an agency's overall mission, the setting of priorities, and examination of the impact of such reductions. In the real world, however, the newspapers were predicting imminent default and fiscal disaster for the city. The Department of Health's response was requested with 24 hours!

Dr. Bellin designated this writer, then the First Deputy Commissioner, to coordinate the requested cuts and to meet with the department's top administrative staff in order to formulate an approach to meet the immediate request. It was decided to absorb the cuts in those services where reductions would have no serious impact on public health.

The senior staff of the department recommended that the 67 positions be cut from the Bureaus of Social Work, Nutrition, and Public Health Education. The staff recommended that a central office nucleus be retained in these three services to serve as a source of expertise for the health districts. The remainder of the personnel reductions came from the elimination of unfilled, vacant budgeted positions. The tax-levy monies reduction was accomplished by reducing funding to the Health Research Council, later eliminated, and by closing three district health centers. Underutilized, their closure had minimal impact.

These initial reductions stirred up a great deal of attention from the press, particularly the cutback in the nutrition program.[12] The degree of this interest, and the pressures placed on the department by groups affected by the reductions, was considerable. As the fiscal crisis continued and even more significant reductions were made in public health services, interest and protest were much less evident, reflecting the understanding that there was no other choice.

FORMULATION OF A RETRENCHMENT POLICY

It was abundantly clear to the senior staff that further budget reductions would be required in 1975 and 1976. Although not yet requested by the city's Office of Management and Budget, it was thought that such requests would inevitably come, and they therefore formulated a comprehensive policy as to how future budget reductions were to be made and which services would be chosen for reduction. This enabled the department to plan for an orderly and well-thought-out retrenchment, and not to respond on an emergency basis to requests from the Office of Management and Budget for cuts.

The department policy included the following three elements:

1) No service would be eliminated entirely. A nucleus would be retained wherever possible.

2) Services were divided into higher priority "life preserving" and lower priority "life enhancing." The former included infectious disease control, and the latter dental public health.

3) Underutilized services and services for which alternative resources existed were to be eliminated first.

While this policy was being formulated, the department set up a liaison structure with the Health and Hospitals Corporation to coordinate service reductions.

In May 1975 the mayor published the crisis budget, which included drastic reductions for most city agencies, and which cut $18 million in tax-levy funds from the Department of Health's budget. At the same time, an austerity budget was also published, which included less dramatic cuts. The crisis budget was not implemented, but budget reductions were required for the austerity budget.[13]

On May 30, 1975 the Office of Management and Budget requested that the Department eliminate 255 positions from specific categories. The department had prepared itself for retrenchment by a policy of setting priorities and minimizing the impact on public health.

The department declined to accept the plan drawn up by the Office of Management and Budget because it did not reflect its priorities. The department drew up a list of 255 positions to be eliminated which reflected its priorities; this was accepted by the Office of Management and Budget. The termination of 255 employees was accompanied by cuts in four programs: Ghetto Medicine, Methadone Maintenance, the Health Research Council, which was eliminated, and the Neighborhood Maternity Center in the Bronx, which was closed (Table 5-2).

In September and October 1975 the Office of Management and Budget asked the department to make a further $3 million reduction in tax-levy funds. This was met by completely cutting all Ghetto Medicine Program monies. Because the state matched these monies dollar for dollar, the risk that the state would also withdraw its funding was serious, but the state agreed to continue its share of the funding without the city doing so.

In addition, the Board of Education removed $970,000 from the School Health Program. This was a major reduction over which the department had no control because the monies for school health are in the Board of Education budget. The impact of this cut, however, was negligible because the department replaced part-time physicians by full-time pediatric nurse-associates and the level of service was maintained.

In July 1976 the last major reductions were implemented, amounting to $4.4 million. In this reduction, district health centers, chest clinics, and child health centers were closed. Dental services, laboratory services, and prison health services were also reduced.

In 1977, this writer, then Commissioner of Health, informed Mayor Beame that no further cuts were possible in the department's

Table 5-2

Reductions in Programs and Clinics, New York City
Department of Health, 1974-1977.

Program/Clinic	Program/Clinic reduction
District Health Centers	7 of 20 closed
Child Health Stations	20 of 76 closed
Dental Health Program	
District Clinics	16 of 27 closed
School Clinics	43 of 164 closed
School Health Program	50,000 of 80,000 physician hours eliminated ($970,000)
Eye Service	14 of 21 clinics closed
Chest Clinics	6 of 14 clinics closed
Tropical Disease Service	1 of 4 clinics closed
Public Health Social Work	10 of 12 social workers terminated
Public Health Education	14 of 19 educators terminated
Public Health Nutrition	18 of 23 nutritionists terminated
Ghetto Medicine Program	$3.3 million reduction (elimination of city support)
Ambulatory Care Program	$1.9 million reduction (elimination of city support)
Health Research Council	Eliminated ($3.3 million)
Bronx Maternity Center	Funding terminated ($600,000)
Methadone Maintenance Program	$1.0 million reduction in budget
Prison Health Service	28% reduction in dental services
	50% reduction in mental health workers (148)
Environmental Health Services	20% reduction in field inspections
Laboratory Services	10% reduction in specimens processed
	Elimination of free vaccines to private physicians

personnel or programs. The department was then suffering the highest attrition rate of any department in city government, due both to retirements and to the flight of younger professionals from New York City. The Mayor and the Office of Management and Budget, alarmed by the high attrition rate, then lifted the hiring freeze, making it possible to recruit a number of young professionals.

PERSONNEL REDUCTIONS

In November 1974 the Department of Health employed 1,600 part-time and 4,400 full-time personnel. During the two-and-a-half-year period following the beginning of the fiscal crisis, the department lost 1,700 people (28.0 percent), and by 1977 had 3,300 full-time and 1,000 part-time employees. Approximately two thirds of this total loss was in full-time personnel, most due not to direct terminations—of which there were about 400—but to attrition from resignations and retirements.

The fiscal crisis demoralized the department. A hiring freeze was imposed in early 1975, no new programs were begun, and existing programs were cut. As a consequence, there was a steady loss of young professionals, managers, and executives.[14]

In July of 1974, 99 executive management positions were filled in the Department of Health. By July 1976 only 60 were filled—a loss of 39 (39.4 percent). This loss of full-time personnel was proportionately greater than the loss of other full-time employees because health executives, managers, and professionals have many employment options, most of which pay competing salaries. Many left the department for more attractive positions.

This attrition was accompanied by the retirement of many pension-eligible employees who feared that their pension eligibility might be jeopardized by the fiscal crisis. Attrition rates for the Department of Health ran, on the average, 60 per month for 1975 and 1976, the highest rate of any department in city government. In large measure, this high rate was due to the exodus of young managers, executives, and professionals.

BUDGET REDUCTIONS

In November 1974 the budget for the Department of Health was $90 million, with $50 million in tax-levy money and the remainder in federal and state grant monies. The state of New York matched the city's tax-levy monies for public health on a 50 percent formula basis. Thus, a tax-levy reduction of $1 was a real program reduction of $2. The total tax-levy reduction in the department's budget was $10 million, part of which is reflected in Table 5-3. This amounted to a 20 percent reduction, from $50 million to $40 million. In addition to the

Table 5-3 Reductions In Personnel And Expenditures In Major
Programs, New York City Department of Health,
1974-1977*

Program	Personnel+ reduction	Expenditure* reduction (tax levy monies)
Administrative and executive	408	847,662
Data center	33	24,244
Public health education	46	209,055
District health services	1,520	3,339,086
Tuberculosis service	14	334,100
Venereal disease services	79	800,000
Total reductions	1,700	5,554,147

*These figures do not include reductions in smaller programs.

+Includes part-time personnel.

major items listed in Table 5-3, $3.3 million was removed from the Ghetto Medicine Program and $1.9 million from the Ambulatory Care Program.

PROGRAM AND SERVICE REDUCTION

Table 5-2 lists the major reductions in programs and services between 1974 and 1977. These cutbacks were implemented to minimize the impact on public health, and some services and programs were either underutilized or outdated. These would have been eliminated eventually, even without a fiscal crisis. In some programs, such as School Health, nurse-practitioners maintained the preexisting level and quality of service at a much lower cost. The closing of district health centers and child-health stations was undertaken with cognizance of alternative facilities, but patients had to travel longer distances for certain services. Some patients did not seek services such as children's immunizations because of increased distances.

Because most of the department's reductions were in the area of life-enhancing services, the impact was not significant for reductions made in 1975. However, the department recognized that life-preserving services could not be reduced or eliminated without serious consequences. Throughout an extremely difficult retrenchment, the department did maintain its life-preserving services intact, and retrenchment of its services had minimal adverse effect on the public health.

PERSPECTIVE ON THE FISCAL CRISIS

The fiscal crisis imposed certain changes on the structure and scope of many departmental programs and functions. Some of these changes were long overdue and would eventually have been implemented even had there been no fiscal crisis. Change is always unpalatable to someone because it results in job loss, frustration of career designs, attrition of bureaucratic domains, and an unsettling of long-established comfortable ways of conducting business. Opposition to change is rarely expressed in these terms. Rather, it is put forth behind such surrogates as the decrying of the discontinuance of allegedly needed services, and the expression of concern over supposed and often imagined consequences.

The Department of Health's retrenchment policy was predictably opposed by various interest groups, from both inside and without. However, the degree of this opposition from within was small, in large measure because broad representation was present from departmental programs and units during the retrenchment effort. Regular weekly and ad hoc meetings were held for almost two years, chaired by this writer and in which all of the deputy and assistant commissioners, as well as managers, participated.

Although the department was smaller after two years of fiscal restrictions, it still retained the quality of its professional leadership and programs. In 1977, the department became part of the city government's Management by Objective Program and was able to hire additional personnel. Life-preserving services were strengthened then, and despite the worst fiscal crisis in the city's history, the department was in a healthy and thriving state.

THE POST-FISCAL CRISIS PERIOD

In the summer of 1976, Bellin informed Mayor Beame of his plans to return to the School of Public Health at Columbia University. He left his position there in 1974 on a leave of absence and had renewed his leave once. In his letter of resignation he strongly recommended my appointment as his successor. This recommendation was supported by Dr. Howard Rusk, Director of the Institute of Rehabilitation Medicine and by Martin Begun, the Associate Dean of New York University's School of Medicine. Both men took an active interest in public health affairs and counseled both Bellin and myself on a number of issues. Their opinion was highly respected by the mayor. In October Mayor Beame announced his intention of appointing me as Commissioner of Health. This appointment took effect January 1, 1977, and carried with it all of the offices occupied by Dr. Bellin, including that of Acting Health Services Administrator.

It is not possible for a Commissioner of Health to render an objective and credible judgment of the quality of his own administration, and I shall not even attempt to do so. It is possible, however, to cite the major issues and problems which arose and to describe the general state of the department. The leading problems and issues which emerged during my fifteen months in office included a major crisis in the HHC that required the removal of the corporations's president, confrontation with the state over the governor's proposal to appoint a city health czar (see Chapter 12), the proposed burn center, the consequences of the blackout that left most of the city without electricity for eighteen hours, the nuclear reactor at Columbia University, sulfur-containing fuels, and the obtaining of young physicians from the National Health Services Corps for underserved areas.

The department's professional staff remained much the same as it had under Bellin's administration, but with some modifications. During 1977 a number of young public health physicians were recruited to replace personnel who had left. Overall, the department was in a healthy state, despite the retrenchment of the fiscal crisis period.

THE KOCH ADMINISTRATION

In November 1978, Edward I. Koch, who had been a U.S. Congressman, successfully defeated Mayor Beame in a three-way contest. He brought to the mayoralty not only dedication and concern, but also a highly individual popularist style. At the time he assumed office, many of the city's fiscal management problems had been rectified.[15] Koch projected a strong and colorful public image that helped restore the faded importance of the mayoralty. But unlike some of his predecessors, he did not generally give his commissioners a free hand to deal publicly with major issues in the press and media, preferring to be the spokesman himself. Unlike Mayors Wagner and Beame, but like Mayor Lindsay, he did not view the Department of Health as exempt from politicization.

Koch was initially intent on revamping the administrative structure for health created during the Beame administration. However, he had not formulated a detailed plan, nor did he perceive that the role of the Department of Health was necessarily separate from that of the HHC. And, as shown by his subsequent policies, he did not assign a high priority to public health.

Prior to his assumption of office, Koch established a search committee headed by his personal physician, a specialist in internal medicine, for the position of Commissioner of Health.[16] The members of this committee forwarded the names of acceptable candidates, my own included. After becoming mayor, Koch reconvened the search committee and requested an expanded search. In the meantime, he asked that I remain in office until he came to a decision. Remaining in office under Koch became increasingly unlikely, not merely because of his clear intention of replacing me, but more important because of his policy toward the Department of Health.

On January 12, 1978 he issued an executive order transferring the powers and responsibilities of the Health Services Administration to the Deputy Mayor for Finance.[17] This meant that the Commissioner of Health was no longer the HHC board chairman although he retained his seat on the board. He then appointed the president of a major voluntary hospital as a "dollar-a-year" special health advisor. And, finally, on March 8, 1978, he issued an executive order appointing a Wall Street investment banker as Special Advisor to the Mayor on Health Services.[18] This individual was also appointed Health Services Administrator, replacing the Deputy Mayor for Finance. The new emerging structure thus included a full-time salaried Chairman of the Board of HHC and a "dollar-a-year" special health advisor. This created fertile ground for potential conflict as the new full-time Chairman of the HHC Board had to define a role for himself somewhere between the functions of the president of the HHC and those of the mayor's "dollar-a-year" advisor.

Against this background, the Health Systems Agency moved to change its bylaws and oust the Commissioner of Health from the de jure right to be either Chairman of the Executive Committee or Chairman of the Board. Groups within both the staff and the board of the Health Systems Agency had always been uncomfortable with this arrangement because it held the potential for significant city control of the agency.

Influencing this change in the bylaws was the situation affecting the executive director of the agency, who was voted into office by the board from an acting position over the objections of the city administration. The objections did not relate to the qualifications of the executive director, but were based on the fact that the board was appointing him without going through the search process required in the agency's federally approved bylaws. The Koch administration unsuccessfully attempted to recommend a search process through its city representatives on the board of the Health Systems Agency.

Shortly thereafter, the board changed its bylaws to enable it and the executive committee to elect their own chairpersons. By so doing, the agency's board perceived that it had divested itself of city control and had achieved the status of a free-standing, independent agency.

In February 1978, I submitted my resignation but agreed to remain in office until March 31. Finally, Koch announced his appointment of Dr. Reinaldo Ferrer as Commissioner of Health. Ferrer, a Puerto Rican public-health physician, had previously held a middle-level position at the Beth Israel Hospital for several years, where he worked under Dr. Ray E. Trussell, the hospital's director.[19] Trussell had a long and distinguished career in public health, having served as Director of the Hunterdon Medical Center in Flemington, New Jersey, Commissioner of Hospitals of New York City, and Dean of the School of Public Health and Administrative Medicine at Columbia University. Ferrer had the qualifications for the commissionership, including a master's degree in public health from Columbia, but he had never filled a high administrative post before. But being from a minority background, over sixty years of age, and willing to allow the mayor to direct public health policy, he had a clear edge over the other candidates. In addition, Herman Badillo, a Congressman of Hispanic origins who had accepted a position with Koch as Deputy Mayor, gave Ferrer's candidacy his full support.

In contrast to what had occurred during the Wagner and Beame administrations, Ferrer accepted a number of political appointees into high executive positions in the department shortly after assuming office. Simultaneously, he made no effort to retain key professionals and vital departmental functions such as drug treatment programs. Additionally, Koch adopted a political policy requiring that all top officials reside within the city. Many officials, including some at the Department of Health, were not prepared to sell their suburban homes and dislocate their families for the sake of insecure positions vulnerable to mayoral whim. The immediate consequences of these policies were a flight of professionals from the department and the loss of programs to state agencies.[20] Ferrer, himself, physically moved out of the office that had been occupied by commissioners since 1935.

In December 1979, one of the department's deputy commissioners, and a political associate of the mayor's, was forced to resign because of his involvement in a milk-dating scandal.[21] A scandal of this kind, involving the department's executive level, had not occurred in over fifty years. Increasingly, the department and the commissioner came under severe criticism.[22] The Committee on Public Health of the New York Academy of Medicine expressed its concern to the mayor over the decline in the professional leadership of the department and the attrition of its functions. The *Village Voice* devoted a front-page story to the department's decline under Mayor Koch.[23] But because public health constituencies are few and not particularly powerful, the criticism and the expressions of concern by the public health establishment had little effect on the mayor, who viewed the department as of minor importance. For there was some political and fiscal advantage for a financially troubled city administration in disposing of costly functions and programs and in not having a strong internal advocate for public health in its midst.

Under Ferrer, the Department of Health rapidly became a lackluster agency, characterized in late 1981 by one highly placed city official as "a forgotten agency of the city." This official added "...It's in real bad shape; The first-rate people are no longer there."[24] According to Deputy Mayor Robert F. Wagner, Jr., the department was no longer in a preeminent position.[25]

Certainly, Koch and his top aides were fully aware of the department's decline well before 1981. Yet they made no efforts to reverse what had become a rapidly disintegrating situation. Removing Ferrer would have been politically hazardous for a mayor facing reelection when his relations with the city's sizeable Black and Hispanic populations were rather poor. Thus, when Ferrer announced in April 1981 that he planned to resign the following September, senior administration officials were not disappointed.[26]

The New York Times, which had remained conspicuously silent about the department's steady decline over a four-year period under Koch and Ferrer, finally published a lengthy article on the subject on October 22, 1981.[27] This paper, which strongly endorsed Koch for reelection three days later on October 25, 1981, never once mentioned Koch's name in the article, nor associated it with the department's decline. Instead, the article, while focusing some blame on Ferrer, gave the erroneous impression that the department had been in decline for decades. This was an unconvincing attempt to take Koch off the hook by spreading the blame far and wide and back over the years. Ferrer understandably defended his four years as head of the department.[28] He focused on the crux of the problem when he said: "A Commissioner of the Department of Health must be above all, loyal to the Mayor."[29] Thus, the favorable environment for decline was created by a mayor who did not assign much importance to public health because of fiscal and political expediency, and by a loyal subaltern who was either unwilling or unable to act as an effective advocate for public health.

By late 1981, the Department of Health had declined to one of the lowest points in its history and had become a public embarrassment for the mayor. The mayor had been acutely embarrassed only a short time before by his choice of Dr. Abraham Kauvar as president of the Health and Hospitals Corporation. Kauvar, who lasted only five months in the position, had been chosen after a nationwide talent search lead by the mayor's chief assistant for health, Victor Botnick, and Deputy Mayor, Robert F. Wagner, Jr., also Chairman of the board of the Health and Hospitals Corporation.[30] Kauvar, who had been head of Denver General Hospital, looked good on paper, but was clearly not up to the demands of the HHC presidency. His removal was finally precipitated by a public comment he made before a group of community and political leaders. Replying to comments on his plans for the as yet unopened Woodhull Hospital, he said, "I think you're looking for a nigger in the woodpile."[31]

These public embarrassments for the mayor, coupled with growing demands for new quality leadership at the Department of Health by the public health establishment, by mid-1981 seemed predictive of a change in direction. In August 1981, the Executive Committee of the Committee on Public Health of the New York Academy of Medicine met with Deputy Mayor Wagner and Victor Botnick to express its concerns about the Department of Health's decline, and the need for appointing an individual of exceptional abilities and qualities as head of the agency. The Committee was told that the mayor would welcome its opinions about the final list of candidates being considered for the post. Koch had by this time set up a search committee consisting of Dr. Saul Farber, Chairman of the Department of Medicine at New York University Medical Center, and Dr. Kevin M. Cahill, a recently appointed member of the Board of Health who had, until late 1980, been Governor Hugh Carey's chief health advisor (see Chapter 12).

By late October 1981, the list of final candidates consisted of Dr. Margaret Grossi, a Deputy Commissioner in the department, Dr. Anita Curran, Commissioner of Health of Westchester County and a former Deputy Commissioner in the New York City Department of Health, Dr. Gilbert Ortiz, a former vice-president of the Health and Hospitals Corporation, and Dr. David J. Sencer, Senior Vice-President of Becton, Dickinson and Company and former Director of the Federal Center for Disease Control in Atlanta. The New York City public health establishment was heartened by this list, as all of the candidates were well-known and respected physicians with extensive public health experience.

During the week of November 22, 1981, members of the New York Academy of Medicine's Committee on Public Health considered the list and undertook an interviewing process. On November 29, Mayor Koch announced his appointment of Dr. David J. Sencer as Commissioner of Health.[32] Sencer's appointment was warmly greeted by the public health establishment and demonstrated that Koch had, to some degree, altered his original low priority policy toward public health. Sencer, who had been Director of the Federal Center for Disease Control for many years, had both a national and international public health reputation and was highly respected for his administrative and managerial abilities.

Chapter 6

STRUCTURE AND FUNCTIONS
OF THE NEW YORK CITY
DEPARTMENT OF HEALTH

Public health services in New York City, as in other local jurisdictions in the United States, derive their authority from the states. This is a product of the Constitution of the United States, and the Tenth Amendment of the Constitution, which permit a sharing of sovereignty between the federal and state governments in matters of health. It reserves for the states powers not delegated to the federal government. Health matters are one of these powers. What has emerged is a sharing of public health responsibilities between the federal government and the states, the latter, in turn, delegating authorities to localities such as cities and counties.

The New York City Department of Health derives its powers from the New York State legislature. That it is a creation of the state has often been forgotten because it has generally functioned in a highly independent manner. This unusual degree of independence for a local health department had its origins in the size of the city and the complexity of its public health problems. Rapid and constant urbanization and waves of new immigrants created a never-ending stream of newer challenges that were alien to the stable rural population of upstate New York. Consequently, the New York State Department of Health had neither the need nor the desire to involve itself in thorny urban health problems. This resulted in a great deal of autonomy for the city's department until the late 1960s, when the state began flexing its muscle with regard to regulatory functions, quality assurance, and standard setting.

STRUCTURE

The New York City Department of Health has long been organized on the scalar principle, which Pfiffner defines as an administrative arrangement consisting of a hierarchy of functional units reporting to a chief executive.[1] Inherent in this principle are the concepts of leadership, delegation of responsibility, and definition of role and function for specific units. Essentially, there is a direct hierarchical line of command from the Commissioner of Health down to each subdivision. Key personnel are responsible to one superior who, in turn, is answerable to the commissioner. The commissioner, in turn, reports to the mayor of the city.

The structure of the department has undergone continuous modification, responding not only to changes in its mission, but also to those in personnel as well. The skills and abilities of those working in the department at any given time have, to a large extent, determined the ultimate form of the organization. Often in the history of the department, form has followed function and not the other way around. Although new programs may have logically belonged in a given unit of the department, they were occasionally placed elsewhere. The reasons for doing this included the perception that the head of the appropriate unit did not possess the necessary skills or motivation to deal with the new program, and the desire to favor another unit head with the program or assignment of the program because of aggressive bidding by a unit head. This, of course, points out one area of frequent breakdown in the scalar principle.

Another frequent area of breakdown in the New York City Department of Health has been in that of internal communications. While the scalar principle holds that all communications must follow hierarchical lines and never short circuit them, the latter frequently occurs, and not necessarily to the detriment of the agency.

The informal organization of the department is, in effect, created by such short circuits. For example, a bureau director may place himself in direct communication with the First Deputy Commissioner, bypassing his immediate superior, a Deputy Commissioner. The short circuiting may be the result of a personal relationship between the First Deputy Commissioner and the bureau director, similarity of professional interest, e.g., both may be epidemiologists, or because of the personalities of the three individuals involved. There are always a number of problems generated by organizational short circuits. However, in the department's history, many of these short circuits have been avoided through the skills of superiors who, aware of their existence, have effectively dealt with them.

THE DEVELOPMENT OF FUNCTIONS

The functions of the department derive from the power and authority granted to it in the city charter.[2] The charter itself is based on powers delegated from the state.[3] As Mustard and Grad have explained, all of these local powers in local health matters are based on the public powers of the state.[3,4]

The health department was once responsible for most public health functions in the city. But after World War II, a number of such functions were assumed by a multiplicity of new governmental agencies, federal, state, and local. In New York State, there were a dozen state agencies that dealt with health matters in 1981, not to mention all of the federal agencies that did. Nonetheless, the department retained responsibility for an enormous spectrum of both preventive and personal services.

There is much diversity in the United States as to how local health departments are organized and what functions they perform.[5] This diversity has been well-documented.[5,6] Succinctly stated, many departments deliver purely preventive services, personal curative services, or combined preventive services and, additionally, engage in measuring and evaluating the quality of medical care and the general health of the population.[7] There has always been much debate about what is appropriate for a local health department, reflecting diverse philosophical points of view. Haven Emerson, a Commissioner of Health of New York City once said that local health departments had six essential functions. These were: communicable disease control, environmental sanitation, vital statistics, maternal and child health, public health education and laboratory services.

During the late 1940s there was considerable expansion beyond these essential six functions within the department. This growth was primarily in the direction of combined preventive services and direct treatment services. The reason for this was the perception that the public health would be furthered by rendering direct services to individuals. A number of eminent public health authorities during the

1940s thought that the new public health frontier was the conquest of chronic diseases. One major avenue of assault was seen in direct treatment services, expecially for the poor who were deprived access because of financial barriers.[8,9] In New York City, health department clinics were often the only resource available to the poor.[9] Miller et al. have cogently argued that health departments must be the last hope of the poor.[10] Their position, based on the premise of equity, is not universally supported. And indeed, some, such as Jonas, have strongly argued against it.[11] The city health department, however, has long held the view that it has both an obligation to render direct treatment services to the poor and that the public health is furthered by approaching certain diseases at the level of the individual. It was because of this commitment and point of view that the department converted 19 child health stations into pediatric treatment centers in 1972.[12]

STATUTORY AUTHORITY OF THE DEPARTMENT

The city charter grants the department specific authority from which derive its functions. In 1975, New York City adopted a new charter. It granted the department jurisdiction to regulate all matters affecting health in the city and to perform all functions and operations that relate to the public health. As stated in the charter, these include, but are not limited to, the following:

enforce all provisions of law applicable in the area under the jurisdiction of the department for the preservation of human life, for the care, promotion and protection of health and relative to the necessary health supervision of the purity and wholesomeness of the water supply and the sources thereof; and shall maintain an office in each borough and shall maintain, furnish and operate in each borough office health centers and health stations or other facilities which may be required from time to time for the preservation of health or the care of the sick;

exercise its functions, powers and duties in the area extending over the city, and over the waters adjacent thereto, within the jurisdiction of the city and within the quarantine limits as established by law;

receive and expend funds made available for public health purposes pursuant to law;

supervise and control the registration of births, fetal deaths and deaths;

engage in or promote health research for the purpose of improving the quality of medical and health care; in conducting such research, the department shall have the authority to conduct medical audits, to receive reports on forms prepared or prescribed by the department; such information when received by the department shall be kept confidential;

supervise the reporting and control of communicable and chronic diseases and conditions hazardous to life and health; exercise control over and supervise the abatement of nuisances affecting or likely to affect the public;

produce, standardize and distribute certain diagnostic, preventive and therapeutic products and conduct laboratory examinations for the diagnosis, prevention and control of disease;

promote or provide education in the prevention and control of disease;

promote or provide diagnostic and therapeutic services for maternity and child health, family planning, communicable disease, medical rehabilitation, narcotics addiction and other diseases and conditions affecting public health;

promote or provide medical and health services for school children and the ambulant sick and needy persons of the city;

promote or provide medical and health services for the inmates of prisons maintained and operated by the city;

maintain and operate hospitals, institutions, public health centers and clinics as shall be established in the department;

prior to the sale, closing, abandonment of a city hospital or transfer of a city hospital to any other hospital or facility, hold a public hearing with reference to such proposed sale, closing, abandonment or transfer; publish notice of such public hearing in The City Record and in such daily newspaper or newspapers published in the city of New York as shall be selected by the commissioner, such publication to take place not less than ten days nor more than thirty days prior to the date fixed for the hearing; and may adjourn such hearing from time to time, if necessary, in order to allow persons interested to attend or express their views;

except as otherwise provided by law, analyze, evaluate, supervise and regulate hospitals, clinics, nursing homes, homes for the aged, clinical laboratories, blood banks, institutions and other facilities providing medical and health services and services ancillary thereto;

supervise and regulate the public health aspects of water supply and sewage disposal and water pollution;

supervise and regulate the public health aspects of the production, processing and distribution of milk, cream and milk products;

except as otherwise provided by law, supervise and regulate the public health aspects of the food and drug supply of the city and other businesses and activities affecting public health in the city;

supervise and regulate the removal, transportation and disposal of human remains;

supervise and regulate the public health aspects of ionizing radiation, the handling and disposal of radioactive wastes, and the activities within the city affecting radioactive materials, excluding special nuclear materials in quantities sufficient to form a critical mass; and

develop, promote, provide, coordinate and evaluate addiction programs for the prevention of addiction and the treatment and rehabilitation of persons addicted to narcotics and other dangerous drugs, including but not limited to the following functions and operations:[13]

> participate in cooperative efforts of federal, state, regional and city agencies and programs dealing with the problems of addiction to narcotics and other dangerous drugs;

> evaluate present and proposed research designs, demonstration projects, treatment and service programs, and other requests related to the prevention of addiction and the care, treatment and rehabilitation of drug addicts in the city, before public funds are made available therefor;

promote or provide research and demonstration projects designed to obtain information relating to the prevention of addiction and the care, treatment and rehabilitation of drug addicts by public or voluntary private agencies supported in whole or in part by city funds;

promote or provide an educational and prevention program to acquaint the public with the problems of addiction resulting from narcotics and other dangerous drugs;

promote or provide treatment modalities for persons addicted to narcotics and other dangerous drugs including but not limited to drug free programs and chemotherapeutic programs, a school based drug prevention program and drug prevention programs and facilities with maintenance of a balance;

annually report to the City Council by March first, as of December thirty-first of the preceding year, on all modalities promoted or provided during the preceding year and proposed to be promoted or provided during the ensuing year with particular reference to the balance between all modalities and the relative effectiveness thereof; and

promote or provide training programs for persons in public or voluntary private agencies and institutions or other facilities engaged in the prevention, treatment and rehabilitation of persons addicted to narcotics and other dangerous drugs.[14]

An Overview of Functions in the 1970s

To some degree, the department is organized to translate these authorities into functions. Functions are grouped into bureaus and divisions and into district services. At the midpoint of the 1970s, there were about 25 bureaus in the department. All administrative services were provided by the Bureau of Audit and Account, while the Bureau of Personnel managed appointments. In addition, there was a Bureau of Maintenance, which dealt with the department's extensive physical plants. The Bureau of Vital Records was responsible for the death, burial, and birth records of the city, while the Bureau of Health Statistics and Analysis compiled city-wide health data and interpreted it. This bureau also conducted analyses of data for the purpose of assisting the commissioner in formalizing public health policies. The Bureau of Child Health operated 78 child health stations and focused on reducing infant mortality and improving child health. Through its day-care center unit, it inspected day-care centers and day camps. The Bureau of School Health supervised school physicians, issued working papers for minor school children, and worked with the Bureau of Nursing and the Bureau of Preventable Diseases in immunizing school-age children.

The Bureau for Handicapped Children offered care and rehabilitation programs to children suffering from visual defects, hearing defects, muscular dystrophy, rheumatic fever, and other handicaps. The Bureau of Dentistry provided dental care for the children of low-income families and educated children in good dental habits at 145 clinics. The Bureau of Public Health Nursing supervised all public health nursing activities. The nurses visited patients ill with communicable diseases in their homes, saw to it that isolation was maintained as prescribed by regulations, took nose and throat cultures, reported on home conditions, advised patients and families as to precautions that should be taken, and generally acted as agents of the department in charge of communicable diseases. In the child-health stations, they assisted physicians and taught mothers how to care for their children. In the schools, they investigated suspicious cases of illness so that the children involved would be examined by the school physician. They also assisted the school physicians in the examination of school children and visited the children's homes to see that the doctor's recommendations were followed.

The Bureau of Nutrition operated nutrition clinics in district health centers and engaged in health education programs. The Bureau of Public Health Education disseminated health information through the media and by publishing pamphlets, circulars, and leaflets. The Bureau of Preventable Diseases was responsible for the department's epidemiological and communicable disease control services as well as for its immunization program. Additionally, it administered a division of veterinary medicine that dealt with the problems raised by forty thousand annual animal bites in the city. Also, the bureau operated four tropical disease clinics that provided free diagnostic and treatment services. The bureau had a staff of both physician and nurse epidemiologists. With regard to the latter, the department instituted a new and unique nurse epidemiology program within the department in the mid-1970s.[15] The bureau also maintained a register of typhoid carriers and worked closely with the Bureau of Food and Drugs in investigating and controlling disease outbreaks. The Bureau of Tuberculosis Control was responsible for all of the department's antituberculosis activities. This included the operation of diagnostic, treatment, and follow-up clinics, and the provision of diagnostic consultation with private physicians. The bureau also supervised cases of tuberculosis at home and worked with the Health and Hospitals Corporation in providing necessary inpatient care. The Bureau of Adult Hygiene was concerned with cancer, mental health, and geriatrics. But by 1974, it was dissolved, as many of its functions were duplicative of those in other governmental and voluntary agencies.

The Bureau of Laboratories managed the various laboratories of the department. It examined milk and food products, shellfish, drinking and harbor waters, cosmetics, and other products. It maintained supply stations in about 400 drug stores and health centers throughout the city, where physicians would obtain diphtheria antitoxin and vaccine, and outfits for forwarding specimens to the laboratories for examination. Such specimens were left at these stations for collection by department messengers.

The Bureau of Food and Drugs investigated and controlled the food and drug supply of the city. The city was divided into districts, each in charge of a supervising inspector. The work involved inspection not only of the foodstuffs, but also of the premises where foods were stored, handled, prepared, and sold. Definite rules and regulations concerning all classes of food stores and factories were enforced by this bureau.

The bureau issued written permits for the sale of milk and monitored the pasteurization requirements of the health code. The Bureau of Sanitary Inspections inspected the 25,000 restaurants in the city as well as stables and slaughterhouses. The major focus of its inspectors, however, was restaurants, because by the mid-1970s, there were only a handful of stables in the city and only one slaughterhouse. The Bureau of Sanitary Engineering dealt with the city's water supply and, in so doing, worked with the Department of Water Resources. It also conducted surveys of the city beaches, assessing them for possible pollution.[16] The Bureau of Radiation Control concerned itself with inspecting and licensing X-ray equipment, and the problems posed by nuclear energy. Its director played a crucial role in formulating the Board of Health's policy of prohibiting the transport of nuclear waster through the city and in preventing Columbia University from activating its nuclear reactor.

The Bureau of Maternity Services, Family Planning and the Newborn dealt with infant care, the welfare of mothers, and conditions and situations in hospital obstetrical services and in nurseries.

The Bureau of Health Care Services supervised medical insurance programs and administered the quality assurance component of the Medicaid Program. It evaluated the quality of services given to Medicaid patients and set standards for their care.

The Bureau of Venereal Disease Control maintained many diagnostic and treatment clinics for the control of sexually transmitted diseases. A staff of public health advisors provided by the Center for Disease Control investigated individual cases and followed up case contacts to insure treatment.

In addition to these functions, the department had a Bureau of Pest Control and a Central Information Service. The latter provided information to telephone callers on a wide variety of inquiries. There was also a Prison Health and Mental Health Service under an Assistant Commissioner. It was responsible for the provision of health and psychiatric services in the city's prisons, which housed approximately 7,000 inmates. The department also operated the New York City Employee Counseling Service, developed by Dr. Hana Rostain, a noted public health psychiatrist. This unit provided screening, referral, and treatment services to municipal employees, with the aim of reducing absenteeism and morbidity due to emotional disorders. Dr. Rostain established a network of counselors throughout most municipal departments and a referral system through which city employees could obtain necessary services.

The department directly operated several methadone maintenance treatment clinics and funded and evaluated close to 30 others. All of these clinics provided services to almost 13,000 patients. With the dissolution of the Health Services Administration in 1977, the supervision and evaluation of free drug programs, previously dealt with by the Addiction Services Agency, were transferred to the Department of Health.

As discussed in the previous chapters that deal with the department's history, bureau functions and categorical activities are carried out not only from a central office, but also from a network of district health centers, child health stations, and school-based clinics. Some direct personal services, such as methadone maintenance, are delivered at sites outside these facilities.

THE CHIEF MEDICAL EXAMINER

In 1967, the Chief Medical Examiner's office was made an agency of the Health Services Administration. However, with the dissolution of the HSA in 1977, the office was placed within the Department of Health as an independent office. The Chief Medical Examiner is appointed by the mayor from the classified civil service list. The city charter provides that the Commissioner of Health not interfere with the performance by the Chief Medical Examiner of his duties nor with his powers.[17] In practice, the Chief Medical Examiner has functioned as an independent agency head with the Department of Health providing supporting services, equipment, and personnel.

MEDICAL AND HEALTH RESEARCH ASSOCIATION

MHRA, as it is widely known, was incorporated in September 1957 as an independent, self-sustaining entity to conduct health research, program evaluations, demonstrations, and pilot studies and service programs for health-related city agencies. These funds are in principle obtained by grant or contract from the federal and state levels and from private foundations. The association is directed at present by a 20-member board of directors.

Although it oversees projects not intimately tied to the New York City Department of Health, the bulk of the association's $12.6 million budget for the fiscal year October 1976 to September 30, 1977 consisted of federal grants given through it to the city Department of Health. During the extremely difficult days of the fiscal crisis in 1975 and 1976, spending and hiring freezes were imposed on all programs, even those funded totally by federal dollars. This policy was later rescinded, but while it was in effect the Department of Health arranged to have a number of such grants channeled through MHRA. An added advantage of this arrangement was the insulation of grants from the city's rather high administrative overhead charges. Most grant monies that MHRA administers are for programs operated by the city Department of Health. Among the most important of these are the Maternity, Infant Care-Family Planning Projects that account for $4.6 million.

Although MHRA has a close operational relationship with the city Department of Health and is from a certain perspective a "fiscal drop" for health department grants, it is administratively quite autonomous. And in recent years it has branched out into activities associated with noncity health-care providers. It is an Article 28 institution, and consequently now has close ties with the state Department of Health.

In late 1981, the Department of Health moved to take direct control of a number of grant programs that had been administered through MHRA. In part, this was in response to altered city budgetary and personnel policies that now made it easier for the department to receive direct funding. Understandably, this move was opposed by MHRA.

Chapter 7

THE BOARD OF HEALTH
AND THE HEALTH CODE

EARLY HISTORY

The first Board of Health in New York City was established in 1805 as an outgrowth of the Health Council that had been created in 1796. The major impetus for its establishment was the 1798 epidemic of yellow fever, which was also the impetus for the creation of the City Inspector's office and the Health Office Commission (see Chapter 2). Of significance is the fact that this first Board of Health derived its authority from the Common Council, which had been empowered to establish it by the state legislature. The board consisted of three state selected commissioners and such others as the council thought appropriate.[1]

The administrative structure for the first half of the nineteenth century was characterized by the existence of three bodies that dealt with public health. The City Inspector was the forerunner of the Commissioner of Health, and was appointed by the Common Council. The Health Office Commission consisted of three state appointed officials. These were the Health Officer of the Port, the Resident Physician, and the Health Commissioner (see Chapter 2). From 1805 to 1823 these three individuals served as ex-officio members of the Board of Health. Thereafter, they were excluded in a successful attempt to eliminate professionals from the board.

As Duffy notes, yellow fever and Asiatic cholera served as the impetus for public health action in the city, with the subsequent creation of the Board of Health.[2] Yellow fever was a serious problem for a thirty-year period, from 1791 to 1821. It served as the major factor in the creation of the Board of Health as well as of the other bodies mentioned above. Yellow fever was seen as susceptible to effective quarantine and, thus, the constant threat of its reappearance served to strengthen the post of Health Officer of the Port, the post which dealt with quarantine. Eventually, however, it was observed that quarantine alone was not successful, and before long the advocates of sanitation made their views known. Their view was that New York's predisposing conditions of dirt and filth were the major factors in spreading both yellow fever and cholera. During epidemic periods, the Board of Health was given emergency powers by the Common Council.[3] When yellow fever struck, it launched city wide sanitary campaigns, imposed strict isolation of cases, built temporary hospitals, provided food and shelter for the sick poor and their families, and on some occasions ordered the evacuation of certain areas of the city.[4]

There were three principal defects in the Board of Health in the early nineteenth century. After 1823, most members were political appointees selected for one-year terms only. And the board was relatively inactive during the long periods when no epidemics threatened the city. This was especially true between the 1821 yellow fever epidemic and the 1832 cholera epidemic. Duffy explains that the Board of Health was extremely slow to respond to the 1832 cholera epidemic, even though it had received sufficient notice because of the disease's rapid spread through western Europe. It was not until a mass exodus of people from the city was underway that the board finally took action.[5] It then began a cleanup of the city and opened several temporary hospitals for the poor. But unlike previous boards, it did not care for the sick poor and their families. It merely solicited private contributions for food and clothing for the poor in cholera hospitals.[6] The slowness of the board's inadequate actions can be explained in part by the fact that it had been inactive for over a decade and was unaccustomed to dealing with health crises. In addition, the board was functioning in a confusing array of health bureaucracies, which resulted in a great overlap of functions. The City Inspector, the Health Officer of the Port, the Resident Physician, and the Health Commissioner all had diverse public health responsibilities, and the latter three functioned as the Health Office Commission. The board's inadequate response was no doubt partially due to its assuming that someone else had matters in hand.

Once the cholera epidemic of 1832 was over, the Board of Health lapsed into an inactive state that lasted until the next cholera epidemic in 1848. According to Duffy, within the narrow confines it had defined for itself, the board functioned reasonably well during the 1848 cholera epidemic. Thereafter, it once again lapsed into inaction.

The real turning point for the Board of Health came in 1866 with the creation of the Metropolitan Board of Health. There were a number of social, economic, and political factors that led to the board's creation (see Chapter 2). The new board aggressively moved to clean up the city on a number of fronts, educate the public, and provide medical care facilities for the sick in the face of an impending cholera epidemic.[8] The epidemic was of limited severity, with full credit going to the new Board of Health. And the board's efforts to clean the city produced visible results much appreciated by the citizenry.

Duffy attributes the success of the Metropolitan Board of Health to the generally high caliber of its officials and staff and to the backing it received from the New York Academy of Medicine and civic reform groups.[9] Blake summarized the board's record when he said it set high standards for energy, scientific talent, vision, and scope.[10] The evidence clearly shows that this board accomplished more in its four-year history than had been accomplished by its predecessors in the previous half century. But the board was part of a reform movement that alienated large vested interests as well as the city's organized Democratic political machine, Tammany Hall. The board itself, in carrying out its missions, had eroded the profits of slum landlords and nuisance trade owners, and had even irritated the medical profession, which resented having to report contagious diseases and other vital data. People quickly forgot the deplorable sanitary conditions that had existed prior to the board's creation and began to focus on the economic costs and the inconvenience of public health measures. But this tarnishing of the glamour of the board's successes did not lead to its abolition. What did was Boss Tweed's gaining control of both the state and city Democratic political machines in 1869. Tweed was able to get a new city charter approved in 1869 which, according to Blake, was specifically designed to make looting the city easier.[11]

In 1870, a new Board of Health replaced the former Metropolitan Board of Health. It was composed of four police commissioners, the Health Officer of the Port, and four health commissioners appointed for five-year terms. As had been the case with the Metropolitan Board of Health, the board was headed by a president, a title that would be retained until 1938, when it was replaced by that of chairman. The title Commissioner of Health was not used in the context of the chief health officer of the city until 1902. It was then that the president of the Board of Health also became Commissioner of Health and head of the Department of Health.

LATER DEVELOPMENTS

In 1873, the first of many modifications was made in the composition of the Board of Health. The board was reduced in size to two health commissioners, the Health Officer of the Port and the president of the Board of Police. The inclusion of police representation is understandable because so many of the Board's actions involved police actions. In 1901, the president of the Board of Police was replaced by the Police Commissioner, who remained a member until 1928, when he was replaced by the Commissioner of Hospitals, a newly created post. The Commissioner of Hospitals remained a member of the board for the next ten years, until 1938. In 1930, the Chairman of the Sanitary Commission became a member, replaced by the Commissioner of Sanitation in 1938.

The year 1938 witnessed major changes in the board's composition because of a new city charter that went into effect. It is noteworthy that between 1901 and 1928 the Board of Health was legally a collective chief executive of the Department of Health. This executive power had its basis in the 1901 city charter.[12] In 1928 an amendment to the City Charter made the Commissioner of Health the chief executive officer of the department. But other provisions of the 1901 charter still gave the Board of Health broad executive powers. In 1938, however, this was altered. The new charter formally gave the Commissioner of Health all the executive power of the board and transformed the latter into a legislative body responsible for the city's Sanitary Code.[13] Given this complicated history, it is understandable why many New Yorkers still view the Board of Health as the operational public health agency of the city and use the name synonymously with the Department of Health.

COMPOSITION OF THE BOARD OF HEALTH

Since 1938, the board has been composed of four members, in addition to the Commissioner of Health who serves as its chairman. This structure has not been altered by subsequent city charters, including the 1977 amendment of the charter concerning the Health Services Administration. The charter requires that two of the four members be doctors of medicine who have had at least ten years' experience in either clinical medicine, public health administration, or college or university public health teaching.[14]

These four members, exclusive of the Commissioner of Health, serve without compensation and are appointed by the mayor for eight-year terms. These terms commence at the expiration of the terms of present incumbents. In the event of a vacancy, the mayor can appoint a member to serve out an unexpired term. The Commissioner designates a full-time Secretary of the Board and other Department of Health employees as may be needed in the board's service.[15]

The mayor may remove a member of the board on proof of official misconduct or negligence in official duties or because of conduct in any manner connected with his official duties that tends to discredit his office. Members may also be removed because of physical inability to perform board duties. Prior to removal, the member is entitled to a copy of the charges, assistance of counsel and a hearing before the mayor.[16]

In December 1981, Mayor Edward Koch sought the resignation of the existing board, an action without precedent in recent decades. In a December 12, 1981 *New York Times* story entitled "Board Reported Asked To Resign," it was reported that Koch had asked the four members to reevaluate remaining through the end of their terms so that a new board could be reconstituted for the city's new health commissioner, Dr. David J. Sencer, who was to take office January 1, 1982 (see Chapter 5).

The Committee on Public Health of the New York Academy of Medicine opposed the mayor's action. It argued that even if the mayor replaced the members with equally qualified professionals, he would establish a dangerous precedent that might permit the future appointment of not-so-qualified individuals. It pointed out that the existing appointment process was a finely tuned mechanism that enabled mayors to replace members as terms expired, but that prevented a given mayor from obtaining board control because terms are staggered.

To many public health professionals in the city, no matter how worthy or appealing Mayor Koch's immediate ends appeared, asking for the board's resignation was no way to achieve them. Many felt that by choosing this route Koch had opened the door to possible future politicization of the board.

The members of the Board of Health have generally been outstanding individuals known for their accomplishments in given fields and in civic affairs as well. Among the physicians who have served on the board over the past fifty years have been two former Commissioners of Health, Dr. Haven Emerson and Dr. Harry Mustard. Other eminent physicians have included Dr. Frank L. Babbott, Jr., once the president of the Long Island College of Medicine, Dr. Thomas M. Rivers, head of the Rockefeller Institute, Dr. Samuel Levine, a noted pediatrician, Dr. Walsh McDermott, a leading public health figure, Dr. Lewis Thomas, president of the Sloan-Kettering Institute, and Dr. Fred Eagle, former Dean of New York Medical College. Nonphysician members have included Paul R. Hays, former head of New York's Liberal Party, and Chester S. Barnard, a distinguished industrialist and former president of the Rockefeller Foundation.

FUNCTIONS OF THE BOARD OF HEALTH

The Board of Health is essentially a legislative body with broad powers that range from issuing permits of different kinds to mobilizing the city's facilities in extreme emergencies in which the life and health of the people are endangered. It grants licences, amends the health code and conducts hearings on important public health issues. The board usually meets once a month, except during the summer, and at such other times as are deemed necessary. Most of the board's actions are related to the Health Code, which is the basis of its power and authority.

THE HEALTH CODE

Section 1706 of the New York City Charter is the source of the power of the Board of Health in regard to the promulgation of the Health Code. Subdivision (2) of this section authorizes the Board of Health to "add to and alter, amend or repeal any part of the code, and may therein publish additional provisions for security of life and health in the city and confer additional powers on the administration not inconsistent with the constitution, laws of this state or with the charter, and may provide for the enforcement of the code or any orders made by the Commissioner or the Board of Health, by such fines, penalties, forfeitures and imprisonment as may be prescribed therein or otherwise by law." The board may include in the Code "all matters and subjects to which the power and authority of the administration extends, not limiting their application to the subject of health only."

Subdivision (4) of Section 1706 provides that "any violation of the Health Code shall be treated and punished as a misdemeanor" and further authorizes civil actions for the recovery of pecuniary penalties for violations of the Code. Subdivision (5) provides that amendments do not take effect until a copy certified by the secretary of the board is filed with the City Clerk. Upon filing, an amendment is to be published in *The City Record*.

Because the authority of the Board of Health in enacting a Health Code is so broadly defined, it has been subject to attack as an improper delegation of legislative authority. In New York, this rule against delegation of legislative authority is based on the provisions of Article 3, Section 1 of the State Constitution, provisions which have been part of the Constitution as far back as 1777 and state that the legislative power shall be vested in the Senate and Assembly. From the very earliest time of the Code (known before the 1959 recodification as the Sanitary Code), however, this delegation of authority to the Board of Health has been upheld in the courts as constitutionally valid.[17] Following these cases, the courts concluded that the constitutionality of this delegation to the Board of Health was no longer in question.

More recently, in a number of cases a new attempt was made to revive this issue of delegation of legislative authority on slightly different grounds. The argument was advanced that a section of the Health

Code (148 Reg. 27) offended Article 3, Section 1 of the State Constitution because the legislature improperly delegated to the Board of Health the power to define certain acts to be criminal offenses. Holding that the Board of Health does not define crimes because the law providing for sanctions is found in the authorizing section itself, 558(d) of the Charter (now 1706(4)), and in 1740 of the Penal Law (now 12-b of the Public Health Law), the court relied on the earlier cases and referred to the Health Code as a "body of administrative provisions sanctioned by the time honored exception to the principle that there is to be no transfer of the authority of the legislature."[18] Recent cases have continued to uphold the delegation doctrine.[19]

There is, however, an exception to an otherwise universal judicial acceptance of the delegation doctrine as it relates to the New York City Health Code: When the code conflicts with existing federal or state law it must yield to such law. Thus, it was held that Health Code provisions requiring the inspection of certain egg products in interstate commerce by a federal inspection service, when inspection by that service is deemed by federal law to be voluntary, intrude on an area of the law already preempted by federal law and which federal law has chosen *not* to regulate.[20] It was similarly held that meat-labelling provisions of the Health Code could not be upheld when such provisions required labelling on products in a manner different from, and in addition to, requirements of previously declared federal and state laws.[21] The Appellate Division, in light of a law giving the federal government exclusive jurisdiction over the labelling requirements in federally inspected meatpacking plants, concluded that federal statutes had already preempted the field as far as interstate commerce was concerned. Similarly, state law had preempted the field in intrastate commerce by means of state regulations that required prior approval before a label might be used on any product prepared under the New York State meat inspection system.

In general, New York City's Health Code contains stricter regulations than the New York State Public Health Law. Because of this, frequent attempts have been made by those affected by various Health Code regulations to have the authority inherent in them transferred to the state. In addition, those subject to regulation are aware that the much longer arm of the state has always been less effective in the enforcement of public health laws than has the city Department of Health.

DEVELOPMENT OF THE HEALTH CODE

New York City's present Health Code developed from early sanitary laws promulgated by Boards of Health in the early nineteenth century. Prior to the advent of the Metropolitan Board of Health in 1866, many of the sanitary laws were never enforced. When they were, such enforcement was sporadic and was carried out during major life-threatening epidemics. Enforcement failure stemmed from the political character of Boards of Health, their relative inaction for long periods of time, and the success of many in obtaining court injunctions against the application of specific sanitary laws. Another factor was the fact that enforcement was in the hands of the police, and the police were not answerable to either the Board of Health or to the City Inspector.

There was a change in this general situation in 1866 when the Metropolitan Board of Health promulgated its new Code of Health. Much in this set of health laws was old, and many doubted that the board would have much success in enforcement. In fact, as Duffy cites, elected judges, concerned about getting votes, continued to issue injunctions on behalf of fat-boiling and rendering plants.[22] Also, these judges had little reason to think that the new board was very different from previous ones that had operated along partisan political lines. Much of the new board's efforts were expended in fighting the injunctions issued by judges. This situation changed, however, later in the year when cholera struck and the board was credited with stopping the epidemic through the application of a broad spectrum of sanitary measures.

In 1870, when the Metropolitan Board of Health was replaced by a new Board of Health, the Code of Health was updated and called the Sanitary Code. Violations of the code were now misdemeanors punishable by fines and imprisonment. Thereafter, changes were continually made in the code, and in time, the Sanitary Code became part of the city's Code of Ordinance. The Sanitary Code was completely revised in 1914.[23] In 1938, however, with the adoption of a new city charter, the Code of Ordinances, which comprised the city's local laws, became the Administrative Code. At the same time, the Sanitary Code became a separate body of law.[24]

In 1955, Dr. Leona Baumgartner, then Commissioner of Health, obtained $100,000 in state and city funds and $60,000 from the Rockefeller Brothers Fund and the W.K. Kellogg Foundation for the purpose of revising the Sanitary Code.[25] Many of the code's provisions were outdated, and mere updating was no longer sufficient. A complete revision was necessary. With these funds Baumgartner entered into a contract with the Legislative Drafting Research Fund of Columbia University to do the actual technical and legal work of rewriting and revising the code.[26] This group began work in October 1955 and produced drafts of various code sections, which were then circulated for comments not only within the Department of Health, but also among a large number of civic and professional groups. The final version of the new code, renamed the Health Code, was adopted by the Board of Health on March 23, 1959.[27,28] Since that time, the code has been constantly updated. As of this writing, the last updated version was published in June 1973.

STRUCTURE OF THE HEALTH CODE

The New York City Health Code is a document some 778 pages long, which is divided into five large title areas and a group of appendices. Title I covers such matters as definitions, the general powers of the department, the Administrative Tribunal, and permit provisions. Title II, entitled "Control of Disease," contains articles dealing with reportable diseases, the regulation of clinical laboratories, the handling of live pathogenic organisms, blood donations and transfusions, blood banks, and artificial human insemination. Title III is entitled "Maternal, Infant, Child and School Health Services." It contains articles dealing with maternity and newborn services, abortion services, nurse midwifery, day-care services, schools and childrens' institutions, and family day-care services. Title IV is an enormous section divided into Part A, which deals with food, drugs, and cosmetics, and Part B, which covers the control of the environment. It contains articles that deal with buildings and commercial premises, drinking water, transportation facilities, insect and rodent control, pet shops, radiation control, hazardous substances, disposal of sewage, littering and refuse disposal, bathing establishments and fumigation. Title V is entitled "Vital Statistics" and contains provisions on the reporting of births, fetal deaths, termination of pregnancy, deaths, the disposal of human remains, and the correction of vital statistics records. The appendices include pertinent sections of the city's charter, those sections of the Administrative Code dealing with the Department of Health and the office of the Chief Medical Examiner, and rules and regulations of the Department of Health.[29]

This overview is by no means an exhaustive coverage of all the articles contained in the Health Code. But it does provide some idea of its comprehensive nature. The enduring quality of this code and its predecessor, the Sanitary Code, is attested to by the fact that segments have frequently been adopted by other states and localities, and even by foreign governments. Although these codes were not intended to serve as ideal models, in point of fact they have because of their inherent qualities and comprehensiveness.

UNIQUE FEATURES OF THE BOARD OF HEALTH AND THE HEALTH CODE

As Baumgartner and Grad have pointed out, the pattern of health legislation in New York City is unique for a locality. As stated earlier, except where Health Code provisions are inconsistent with the constitution and laws of the state, the Board of Health constitutes the final legislative authority on health matters in the city.[30] In addition, the authority of the board is not limited to health matters alone, but extends into all areas subject to the authority and powers of the Department of Health.[31] Thus, the board has been given broad legislative powers, and the Health Code constitutes a unique document. As mentioned above, both the board's authorities and the legality of various provisions of the code have been challenged frequently in the courts.

Baumgartner and Grad make a cogent point in saying that in some municipalities the promulgation of a health code is essentially the task of a City Council. In other municipalities, a health code is enacted by the Board of Health, subject to further approval by a City Council.[32] In this model, health commissioners often promulgate regulations administratively. There are many variations on these patterns.[33]

The Board of Health in New York City is, in effect, a small legislature dealing with public health matters from the position of a broad mandate. City charters have not given health commissioners powers to promulgate general regulations other than those dealing with internal management matters within the Department of Health. Consequently, the Health Code of 1959 was written to allow for proper public health administration, yet retain a flexibility that would avoid the need for constant amendment changes needed to deal with minor public health practice changes.[34]

LEGAL SERVICES

Because the Board of Health has such sweeping legislative powers and authorities over health matters in the city, and because the Department of Health is responsible for the enforcement of code regulations dealing with public health, the department has long had a Legal Division. During the 1970s, this division was headed by a General Counsel who was the counsel to both the Board of Health and the Department of Health. The division was staffed by several lawyers as well.

Both the board and the department were fortunate in the 1970s in having two successive General Counsels with extensive experience and training in public health law. Harry Hollander, who served as General Counsel for many years, was succeeded in 1975 by Irving M. Witlin, who, in addition to being an attorney, had also served as a sanitary inspector in the department and held a masters degree in public health from Columbia University. Both men were extremely knowledgeable, not only about the Health Code, but also about the multiplicity of other local, state, and federal laws dealing with public health matters. Their tenures coincided with a period of expansion of the department's standard setting and medical care regulatory functions and with newer complex environmental health issues.

Chapter 8

THE CHIEF EXECUTIVE

Although the chief executive, in this instance the Commissioner of Health, heads an agency containing many professional peers and colleagues, he or she ultimately sets the tone for the agency. Excellence replicates itself just as does mediocrity. In the final analysis, it is the Commissioner of Health who usually chooses the deputy, associate, and assistant commissioners and, in so doing, meets his own established standards, whatever they may be.

The selection of commissioners of health by incoming mayors was not institutionalized as a nonpolitical process devoid of the influence of partisan politics until 1926, when the accumulated abuses of eight years of Tammany Hall led to a change in this political machine's attitude toward the Department of Health. Their successful candidate, Mayor James Walker, promised to take politics out of the department, a promise he kept.

Prior to this time, a number of commissioners were chosen on the basis of professional merit, but a sizeable number were also selected because of their partisan political loyalties. This was especially true during the eight-year period between 1918 and 1925. All three physicians who served during this time as Commissioner of Health were closely associated with the ruling Democratic Party, and one was also the mayor's private physician.

SELECTION PROCESS

The growth of public health as a distinct medical specialty requiring specific skills to deal with increasingly complex problems served as a deterrent to mayoral selection of personal physicians and politically loyal physicians lacking training and experience. Physicians with strong partisan political convictions rarely had this kind of training and experience and, during the past half century, only one public health physician with partisan political connections has been appointed Commissioner of Health.

Public health has not been a high-income specialty for physicians in recent decades. Consequently, politically connected physicians have not been attracted to it out of motives of financial gain. Also, professional peer groups such as the New York Academy of Medicine have exerted great influence on mayors in requiring high performance standards of health commissioners. This confluence of positive influences created an environment that was scarcely comfortable for a commissioner lacking in qualifications. And indeed, in time, specific experiential and training qualifications for the post were written into the city's charters. Among these are that the individual must have an M.D. degree, eight years of public health experience, and an M.P.H. or equivalent degree.[1] Generally, the enforcement of these criteria by outside watchdog groups has been intense. For example, in 1946 Mayor O'Dwyer was obliged to rescind the ten-day-long appointment of Dr. Edward N. Bernecker because he did not have an M.P.H. or equivalent degree. Bernecker was a superb administrator and had served as Commissioner of Hospitals. Still, watchdog groups demanded his removal because he did not have the legal qualifications for the job.[2] Of note, however, is the fact that there was no such outcry twenty years later when Mayor Lindsay appointed Dr. Howard Brown as Health Services Administrator and Commissioner of Health. Like Bernecker, Brown did not have an M.P.H. degree, but was qualified for the health commissionership in every other way. Part of the reason for no protest was the fact that Brown was primarily appointed Health Services Administrator and was given the health commissionership for eight months as a temporary arrangement (see Chapter 3).

City charter qualification requirements have served as a strong deterrent to the appointment of nonprofessionals and unqualified individuals to the health commissionership. They do not, however, prevent the appointment of qualified physicians with partisan political loyalties and connections. But, in point of fact, only one such individual was appointed during the period 1930-1980. There has always been more jeopardy than gain for mayors in trying to downgrade the qualifications for the commissionership.

The selection of health commissioners in New York City by mayors according to charter standards and often through professional search committees is at variance with the way in which commissioners of a number of other departments are chosen. Commissioners of some city departments are often chosen because of their preelection loyalties. Others, however, such as those in the Fire and Police Departments are frequently professionals with neither political affiliations nor loyalties. This heterogeneity of the selection and appointment processes is not generally perceived or understood by the casual observer. Thus, those who term all commissioners of health as "politicians" or "political appointees" do so out of ignorance.

As shown in Table 8-1, of the eighteen health commissioners who served between 1924 and 1982, nine (50 percent) were individuals who had already served in the Department of Health and nine (50 percent) came from outside the department. In addition, Philp, who was Acting Commissioner, had been First Deputy Commissioner, and Bushel, who succeeded him as Acting Commissioner of Health, had been a deputy commissioner. Margaret Grossi, who served briefly in 1981 as Acting Commissioner, had previously been a deputy commissioner. Of note is the fact that of the nine insiders appointed, six had been either deputy or first deputy commissioners. Between 1969 and 1981, four first deputy commissioners became Commissioner of Health. This position is filled, according to the New York City Charter, by an individual who has the same qualifications as the Commissioner of Health. In some instances, commissioners have groomed their first deputies to succeed them.

Table 8-1
Commissioners of Health, New York City, 1926-1982

Name	Tenure	Position from Which Appointed
Louis I. Harris	1926-1928	Director, Bureau of Preventable Diseases
Shirley W. Wynne	1928-1933	Deputy Commissioner
John L. Rice	1934-1942	Commissioner of Health, New Haven, Connecticut
Ernest L. Stebbins	1942-1946	Professor of Epidemiology Columbia University

Table 8-1 (cont.)

Edward M. Bernecker	1946	Commissioner of Hospitals
Israel Weinstein	1946-1947	Director, Bureau of Public Health Education
Harry S. Mustard	1947-1948	Director, School of Public Health, Columbia University
John F. Mahoney	1949-1953	Director, USPHS Venereal Disease Laboratory
Leona Baumgartner*	1954-1962	Assistant Commissioner, Maternal and Child Health
George James	1963-1965	Deputy Commissioner
John Philp (Acting)	1965	First Deputy Commissioner
Arthur Bushel (Acting)	1966	Deputy Commissioner
Howard Brown	1966-1967	Director, Ambulatory Care, Gouverneur Hospital
Edward O'Rourke	1967-1969	U.S.P.H.S.
Mary C. McLaughlin	1969-1972	First Deputy Commissioner
Joseph A. Cimino**	1972-1974	First Deputy Commissioner
Lowell E. Bellin***	Jan. 1974-Jan. 1977	First Deputy Commissioner
Pascal James Imperato	Jan. 1977-March 1978	First Deputy Commissioner
Reinaldo A. Ferrer	April 1978-Sept. 1981	Associate Director, Professional and Academic Affairs Beth Israel Hospital
Margaret Grossi (Acting)	Sept. 1981-Jan. 1982	Deputy Commissioner
David J. Sencer****	Jan. 1982-	Vice-President, Becton Dickinson and Company

---

*Dr. Baumgartner had resigned from the department in April 1953 to become Director of the New York Foundation.

**Dr. Cimino served as First Deputy Commissioner for only a few weeks. Prior to that he had been Director of Health and Safety, New York City Environmental Protection Agency.

***Dr. Bellin resigned from the department in early 1972 to become Professor and Head of the Division of Health Administration, Columbia University, School of Public Health.

****Dr. Sencer served for several years as Director of the Federal Center for Disease Control in Atlanta, Georgia.

Mayors have often formed search committees to screen candidates for the commissionership. But they have not always bound themselves to the recommendations of these committees. Other mayors have chosen commissioners of health on the recommendations of respected medical authorities, and some have used a combination of these methods. Rarely, since the enactment of charter requirements for the commissionership, have mayors made a choice on the basis of advice or pressures from political associates or political clubs. Even if a mayor made an appointment in response to these pressures or advice, the candidate would still have to meet the charter requirements.

Mayoral choice of a health commissioner has also been strongly influenced by what is desired of the person in the position and of the department in general. Mayors such as La Guardia, Wagner, and Beame, who adopted a policy of leaving public health matters to professionals, chose health commissioners of the highest quality. They also allowed their health commissioners to make all departmental appointments. Other mayors, such as O'Dwyer, Lindsay, and Koch, had less consistent policies, appointing some excellent health commissioners because of professional merit and following a hands-off policy and others in order to bring the department into line with larger administration political goals. Strong health commissioners demand a fair share of the city's operating budget, speak up on behalf of public health issues, and vigorously protect their department's functions and resources. This is not the type of health commissioner usually desired by financially strapped administrations or by strong, dominating mayors.

Mayors Wagner and Beame chose an option that is a mixed blessing for an elected official. On the one hand, they were comfortable in the knowledge that highly complex and volatile health-care problems were in the hands of professionals. On the other hand, they knew that the professionals' loyalty could not be counted upon if it came into conflict with allegiance to professional standards.[3] In other words, the professional's loyalty to a politician is never completely reliable. This is an accommodation these mayors made in return for commissioners who demonstrated strong leadership and a willingness and ability to assume visible responsibility for dealing with difficult problems and implementing unpopular solutions. Both these two mayors and some others who chose top professionals as health commissioners found themselves in conflict with their appointees on a number of occasions. For their health commissioners placed loyalty to professional standards above fidelity to the political administrations that appointed them. Some mayors, uncomfortable with this situation, sought to prevent or correct it by appointing professionals who were not strong leaders and who were willing to allow them to formulate public health policy.

DISMISSAL

All city commissioners, including those of health, serve at the pleasure of the mayor. Therefore, they can be dismissed by the mayor at any time. Of the eighteen health commissioners who served between 1928 and 1982, nine (50 percent) resigned voluntarily, eight (44.4 percent) were forced to resign, and one is still in office. Commissioners have frequently resigned just before the end of a mayoral term, and a few have resigned during a term. Resignations just before the end of an outgoing mayor's term or coincident with it have been prompted mainly by the knowledge that with the exception of Dr. John F. Mahoney, who served both Mayors O'Dwyer and Impelliteri, no recent Commissioner of Health has successfully bridged a change in the city's administration. Some commissioners have stayed on into the early months of a new mayor's term to assist in an orderly transition, but with the understanding that they would shortly resign. Others have remained on with the hope of reappointment, and when it was clear that this was not going to occur, have resigned. In the former instance, the resignations have been voluntary and, in the latter, forced. As the historical facts show, mayors prefer to appoint their own commissioner of health and except for Mayor Impelliteri, have not retained holdover commissioners. Voluntary resignations during a mayoral term have been prompted by a desire to retire, illness, the need to return to a position from which a leave of absence was taken, and the offer of a better position.

Forced resignations during a mayoral term have occurred on four (22.2 percent) occasions since 1928. In one instance, the appointee did not have the qualifications for the position.[4] But in the remaining three there were mayor-commissioner conflicts over policy issues. Thus, in recent years, the ratio of the risk to commissioners of forced resignation over policy has been close to one in four.

SELECTION OF DEPUTIES

City charters have spelled out the number of deputy commissioners who may be appointed. The most recent charter calls for four deputy commissioners, one of whom must have the same qualifications as the commissioner and one who shall be responsible for the drug treatment and prevention programs authorized by law.[5] The former has been called the first deputy commissioner and has frequently been assigned major responsibilities for departmental operations. Commissioners have often given the title deputy commissioner or associate commissioner to individuals who have actually filled lines budgeted at the assistant commissioner level. These individuals have often been referred to as "paper deputies" by departmental insiders, signifying that the title is a departmental one.

Most commissioners have chosen their deputies, and mayors have approved their selections. Occasionally, mayors have forced appointments on commissioners in either an attempt to reward preelection loyalties, or to gain some degree of control over the department or both. Strong commissioners have successfully resisted such attempts, and some mayors, such as Wagner and Beame, never even engaged in them. Clearly, a commissioner who does not choose his own deputies is not in complete control of the department. And indeed, this has been borne out in those instances when mayorally chosen deputies have moved into the department.

Deputies serve at the pleasure of the commissioner and can be removed at will. Since deputies are often chosen from among departmental professionals, they often have a civil service line to which they can return if removed from the higher position. This has rarely occurred, as most deputies have served throughout a commissioner's term and have usually moved on to positions outside the department at the end of that term. Some deputies have continued on into the term of a new commissioner, but this has not occurred with any great frequency. What has been more usual is the continuance of bureau directors through the terms of successive commissioners. Their continuance, and that of district health officers and other staff, is what has provided the department with professional continuity.

OTHER FUNCTIONS

Although one previous Commissioner of Health under Lindsay had served simultaneously as Health Services Administrator, none had also served as Chairman of the Board of Directors of the New York City Health and Hospitals Corporation (HHC). Beame coordinated all of the city's health activities in the person of the Commissioner of Health. His two commissioners were simultaneously Health Services Administrator, Chairman of the Board of HHC, and Chairman of the Executive Committee of the Health Systems Agency of New York City. This gave the Commissioner of Health a number of major responsibilities outside the Department of Health. As Chairman of the Board of the HHC, the Commissioner of Health was the chief officer of a system composed of 17 municipal hospitals with 8,000 beds and 35,000 employees. The annual operating budget of the HHC was $1.2 billion. Although the HHC had a president and a staff responsible for operations, the board formulated policy and decided on a number of key issues.

In addition to chairing the Board of the HHC and representing the views of the city administration on it, the Commissioner of Health was also Chairman of the Executive Committee of the Health Systems Agency. This committee then had authority under the law to review and approve or disapprove a wide range of capital expenditures proposed by institutional health-care providers and pass its actions on to the full board of the Health Systems Agency for approval. This position gave the Commissioner of Health a key role in the health-planning process and established a conduit for input from the staff of the Department of Health.

In recent years, commissioners have also been ex-officio members of a number of boards and committees of nongovernmental bodies such as the Community Council of Greater New York, the Greater New York Hospital Association, the Committee on Public Health of the New York Academy of Medicine, the Medical Health and Research Association, and the Public Health Research Institute. Membership in these groups consumes a great deal of time, and for this reason, commissioners have had to either delegate a departmental member to represent them or have had to delegate departmental functions so that they can devote meaningful time to these other organizations.

RELATIONS WITH THE MAYOR AND DEPUTY MAYORS

A commissioner functions in a larger government bureaucracy. Even though he reports directly to the mayor, in practice, mayor-commissioner contacts are usually limited to very important matters, and such contact is often by telephone. Although commissioners attend monthly mayoral cabinet meetings, weekly contact with City Hall is maintained through the deputy mayor, who has been delegated health affairs as an area of concern. Contact is also maintained through mayoral aides and aides to the deputy mayor just mentioned. A commissioner either knows or learns very quickly that mayors do not have the time or attention span to become involved in any but the most crucial issues. And in New York City there have been only a few such issues per year. In most cases, commissioner-mayor contacts usually consist of the former briefing the latter. Decision making usually rests with the commissioner and his staff.

The interactions of a commissioner of health and a deputy mayor whose concerns include health vary in intensity with the person occupying this appointive office and the issues at hand. It would be a naive chief executive of a public health agency who failed to realize that individuals in such offices have political aspirations of their own. Thus, their views may not necessarily reflect those of the mayor, and they and their assistants not infrequently invoke mayoral authority and convey mayoral wishes without the mayor's knowledge. A commissioner must also recognize that mayors may attempt to exert influence over professional decisions through immediate subordinates and particularly through the staff assistants of such subordinates. He must be capable of resisting such influence even to the point of confrontation if it would result in a breach of professional integrity. He must also recognize that resistance to such interference usually serves as a warning to superiors who will think twice before trying it again. Another key point not to be forgotten is that some mayoral or deputy mayoral efforts to influence are only posturing exercises. There is no serious desire to alter a decision; the only objective is to enable the mayor or deputy mayor to say to the advocacy group initiating the attempt that he did his best. In this way, an elected leader does not alter a sound professional decision that is not in the best interests of a loyal support group, nor does he lose their loyalty.

RELATIONS WITH SUBORDINATES

A commissioner must also deal with his own staff. To be successful, he must not only choose staff who are well-trained and experienced, but must also delegate sizeable responsibility to them. Failure to do either insures the commissioner's own failure. Staff take their cues from their leader and learn quickly what is expected of them. A commissioner must realize that each key staff member is an advocate for his or her programs. It should hardly surprise him that the assistant commissioner for maternal and child health, while agreeing to the importance of chronic disease programs, argues that dollars are better spent on mothers and children than on glaucoma screening.[6] Programs are, in a sense, surrogates for those who direct them. It is evident, therefore, that in a pyramidal organization, professionals compete for the higher positions by advocating policies and programs with which they are identified. Career success is perceived as being intimately linked to program success.

In dealing with his staff, the commissioner must initially institutionalize the process in which delegated responsibilities are discharged by those to whom they are entrusted. Subordinates often tend to shift the responsibility back to a superior. Instead of stating the problem and recommending solutions, they merely state the problem, hoping the commissioner will formulate the solution. If the latter is unwise enough to do so, he has, in effect, assumed the task of his subordinate. During Beame's administration all administrative layers in the New York City Department of Health clearly understood that recommended solutions were expected of them. This practice, coupled with the delegation of the daily operating responsibilities of the department to a first deputy commissioner, enabled the commissioner to fulfill his numerous obligations.

In order to retain good staff, a commissioner must be sensitive and responsive to the needs of individual departmental leaders. Deputy, associate, and assistant commissioners must be encouraged and rewarded if morale is to be maintained and if they are to be retained by the department. Within the general policy goals of the department, and as permitted by fiscal resources, the commissioner must give his support to his key personnel for the department to run successfully. These key personnel must, in turn, be sensitive and responsive to the needs of their subordinates and also support them.

Chapter 9

ESTABLISHING PRIORITIES

The New York City Health Department provides a wide range of services and programs. Each of these has its internal advocates within the department as well as a number of external ones. Among the latter are the beneficiaries of specific programs, the professionals, paraprofessionals and workers on the payroll of such programs, members of governing committees of programs, indirect beneficiaries such as unions of health workers, and the ideological supporters of programs.[1] All of these groups can persuasively argue high prioritization of their programs with both sincerity and supporting data. They also denigrate, usually in less candid language, other programs, inferring they have a much lower priority. Deciding on the prioritization of specific programs is a complex process in which subjective professional values, political process, knowledge of the health status of the population, and the application of economic measures to outcomes play a role. Often, the impetus to either shrink or expand programs is fiscal.

THE INFLUENCE OF HEALTH STATUS

Health status determination is a difficult process. Data are usually generated through population surveys, census taking, and prevalence reported to local and state health agencies. Health status is often inferred from demographic information, particularly in situations where there is a strong relationship between age, sex, income level, or ethnicity, and specific diseases or medical problems.[2] But such determinations are affected not only by errors inherent in the sample survey techniques usually used to obtain the data, but also by the inferential process as well.[3]

Schonick points out that health service needs cannot simply be determined by knowledge of the health status of the population because of the division of professional opinion about the benefits of certain preventive, diagnostic, and therapeutic measures.[4] This is certainly true of a number of surgical measures, such as coronary bypass surgery, tonsillectomy, and radical mastectomy. It is less true for many of the personal services provided by a health department, such as childhood immunizations, dental services, and sexually transmitted disease therapies.

Many health department services have evolved over the decades in large measure because of the choices, based on an objective reading of morbidity and mortality data, made by professionals. Dramatic results have been demonstrated when interventions have been aimed at certain types of disease problems such as the communicable ones. However, intervention outcome is much more difficult to assess with chronic conditions because positive results often consist of pain alleviation and improved function, but not disappearance of the disease.[5]

Wants

Specific groups may want a particular service for a variety of reasons. However, their common link is often that of self-interest. Disease sufferers want it because it helps them. Unions and workers want it because it provides jobs. Professionals want it because it provides a place for their skills. And finally, communities may want it because it adds a desired dimension to their lives. The wants of various groups may or may not positively correlate with the need for specific health services as objectively determined by an analysis of available data. However, wants can and do generate demands for services that are often channeled through the political process. Consumer groups and citizen groups, for example, are often well-organized to have wants met. And, in recognition of the legitimacy of wants, consumers are frequently on the boards of hospitals and other health facilities.[6]

Needs

Needs can be determined to a certain extent by an examination of morbidity and mortality data and of data generated by special surveys. Needs can also be determined by the opinions of experts based on an examination of a spectrum of facts and data. In general, it is easier to estimate needs than wants and, consequently, professionals usually act to create programs to meet these needs if deemed necessary.

DEMAND, USE AND SUPPLY

Demand represents want modified by factors such as cost in financial terms and patient effort. Since the public health services provided by the New York City Department of Health are free, modifiers such as travel cost and time often reduce demand to a quantitative level below that of want. However, it is still difficult to measure demand except through special sample surveys.

On the other hand, it is relatively easy to measure use or utilization of personal services because data are available for all of the department's clinics. In the department's recent history, it has been found that when there is a strong correlation between want and need, there is a similar correlation between these two elements and use.

The supply of public health facilities providing various services in recent times in New York City has generally been adequate to meet both needs and demands. However, at various points in time they may not have met wants. Often, need has been greater than demand, as when accessible and available free services are not utilized by the inner city poor.

ECONOMIC MEASURES

Health economists are frequently called upon to quantify the worth of public health programs. One of the measures they use is the supplementary earning power that can be achieved by the beneficiary of public health intervention.[7] Some think that this results in more objective decisions about prioritization. However, as Bellin points out, this process merely operationalizes a specific social value. This enhances the premise that productivity, financial independence, and the ability to pay taxes by the foetus whose health is preserved are to be cherished over the alleviation of the physical and mental discomfort of elderly nonearners.[8] Other societies in other places and other times made different choices, viewing the elderly as sages precious to the maintenance of the wisdom of the culture.[9]

When all is said and done, economic measures do not have unique impact on allocative decisions. Nor for that matter do objective data. What does is a combination of subjective values which operate within complex political processes and which are influenced to some degree by objective data, needs, wants, and economic measures.

THE ROLE OF POLITICAL PROCESS

Bellin points out that although the data concerning health status may be clear-cut, their salience may not be so to the public, to constituencies, to the spokesmen who purport to represent the constituencies, to elected and appointed officials, and to public health professionals.[10] He cogently notes that the salience of the data changes as the perceptions of the data change, as the values change, and as the times change.[11] He uses the example of the perception of three deaths from diphtheria among children per annum in 1900 as a blessing. The same number of annual deaths in New York City in the last quarter of the twentieth century would be perceived as a catastrophe.[12] One could also say that ten times that number of deaths in the city from automobile accidents would cause little excitement.[13] Thus, perceptions of the data are greatly influenced by the times and the preventive armamentarium of the times. It is really the political process that finally determines what social value is turned into a public health program.[14] This process involves the interaction of various groups, including the advocates of a program within the Department of Health, clientele-beneficiaries of the program, the professionals, paraprofessionals, and workers on the payroll of the program, the members of advisory or governing boards of the program, the indirect beneficiaries of the program, including unions and merchants within the catchment area of a health facility, and the ideological supporters of health programs.[15] All of these groups predictably support the enhancement and resist the shrinkage of the health program of interest to them.

Single-issue constituency was a growing phenomenon in the U.S. during the 1970s. Both elected and appointed leaders were often judged by constituent groups, not on the basis of their overall performance, but rather on whether or not they enhanced the single-issue constituency's program.[16] Such groups engage in hyperbole to enhance their program and use a variety of pressure tactics aimed at achieving programmatic enhancement. In addition, some have been successful in pressuring legislative bodies to mandate their programs. These mandated programs are the most resistant to dismantling once the need for them has passed, because this invariably requires protracted legislative action.

MANDATED PROGRAMS

Most mandated programs administered by the New York City Department of Health have come into being not because of single-issue constituency strategies, but rather because there was a perceived need for them. Some have arisen from the legislative action of the Board of Health, others from laws passed by the City Council, and yet others from laws passed by the state legislature.

In rare instances, public health programs have been mandated without the provision of enforcement resources. An example of this type of program is the dog litter ordinance passed by the New York City Council in 1978. This law came into being after it had been introduced in committee for many years by city councilmen who advocated its passage. In addition, there were a number of advocacy groups that had pressed for the law. The crucial issue that the law attempted to address was the aesthetic problem of dog feces and urine, particularly in high-density middle-class neighborhoods such as the upper east side of Manhattan. But in its support this proved to be a weak argument. Advocates then pushed forward the argument that dog litter on the streets and in the parks was a major source of visceral larva migrans, a systemic disease caused by the migrating larvae of a nematode, *Toxocara canis*. Since this disease primarily affects children, this argument had great appeal.

The Department of Health, however, disputed the prevalence data on visceral larva migrans presented by advocates and pointed out that most cases were contracted by children having domiciliary contact with infected puppies. The disease is most prevalent in puppies, and infection rates fall off sharply in dogs over one year of age. Departmental professionals argued that the more serious problem was that of dog bites, of which some 40,000 were then being reported annually in the city.[17] In effect, the department argued that the council was focusing its attention on the wrong end of the dog.

   As the legislation was being formulated, the council attempted to delegate enforcement to the health department. Because the professional consensus in the department held that dog litter was primarily an aesthetic problem and not a public health one, the department successfully fought against its designation as the enforcing agency. Consequently, policemen, traffic enforcement officers, and Department of Sanitation inspectors were given enforcement responsibility. This diffusion of the responsibility, coupled with the fact that no additional manpower resources were provided, almost guaranteed low enforcement levels. Indeed, because of the city's fiscal crisis, the ranks of those required to apply the law were reduced. Yet, some citizens did comply and purchased "pooper-scoopers" or else cleaned up after their animals had defecated. But this public spirited minority did not offset the net effect of the majority who ignored the law.

Chapter 10

THE BUDGET

Because of its size and the comprehensiveness of services provided by the city, New York's municipal budget is unique.[1] The annual budget consists of two parts, the expense budget and the capital budget. The latter is actually the city's capital improvements spending plan for large equipment purchases and new facilities.[2] In recent years, the capital budget has been financed from borrowings. However, from the beginnings of the fiscal crisis in 1975 until the early 1980s, there have been few expenditures made out of the capital budget.

The expense budget is the city administration's plan for financing daily operations. It reflects a host of policy decisions, political processes involving competing constituencies, and the administration's obligation to support mandated programs. In theory, the city's expense budget is supposed to be financed from current revenues. However, in practice it was often financed from borrowings and out of the capital budget. In the latter instance, expense budget items were placed in the capital budget (see Chapters 1 and 5).

HISTORICAL BACKGROUND

As is the case in many large, centralized, governmental bureaucracies, New York City's government has long had a Bureau of the Budget. This unit was originally under the control of the city comptroller, later under the Board of Estimate, and has more recently become part of the mayor's office. Because of flagrant spending abuses, reformers set up a system of controls which culminated in the 1938 charter revision under Mayor La Guardia. This charter transferred the Bureau of the Budget from the Board of Estimate to the mayor's office, but required that budget schedules be approved by the board. The bureau, now known as the Office of Management and Budget, continued to exercise line item controls, effectively imposing elaborate processing requirements on city agencies. While the original intent of these controls was good, namely to thwart abuse, they eventually assumed proportions that made them destructive burdens. In an attempt to ease these burdens, the 1963 charter introduced units of appropriation into the budget and eliminated the Board of Estimate's authority over schedule changes.[3] The Bureau of the Budget, however, in a successful stroke of bureaucratic power was able to maintain the status quo by invoking other requirements of the charter.[4] The 1975 charter attempted to eliminate many of the administrative controls exercised by the Office of Management and Budget, but was unsuccessful. And for the remainder of the 1970s, the fiscal crisis became the reason for their continuance.[5]

The elaborate controls built into the budgeting process in New York City, while instituted to prevent overspending and abuse, have often resulted in the creation of unnecessary obstacles to launching new programs, hiring new personnel, and even getting hired personnel on the payroll. For example, in the 1970s it required an average of six months from the time a new health department employee started work until they received their first paycheck. In order to deal with this problem, the department had to set up a system of interest free loans from a special charities fund that had been created by employees. Later, when this fund was exhausted, the comptroller set up a fund of fifteen thousand dollars to deal with the problem.[6]

UNITS INVOLVED IN THE BUDGETING PROCESS

New York City possesses an elaborate budgeting process that involves various governmental units. The comptroller is responsible for collecting revenues and for auditing expenditures to ensure that they are being made in accordance with the codes of the budget. The

Office of Management and Budget is responsible for drawing up the city's budget on an annual basis, in concert with various city agencies. The Board of Estimate, consists of the mayor, the comptroller, and the five borough presidents, must approve the budget before it is adopted, as must the City Council, which is a legislative body.

The Department of Health, like most city agencies, possesses units that deal with management and budget. During my administration, these functions were directed by a superbly qualified Deputy Commissioner for Administrative Services, Louis Neugeborn. Under his direction were seven offices key to the budgeting process. These included: fiscal affairs, budget administration, personnel and labor relations, electronic data processing, management audits and investigation, general services, and management information reporting.

THE BUDGET-MAKING PROCESS

Fiscal policy is largely determined by the decision-making processes that take place within the department (see Chapter 11). Once this policy is established, a long and arduous process takes place within the department to establish a budget. The process continues in concert with the Office of Management and Budget until the final budget is ready for submission to the Board of Estimate and the City Council.

As Bellin has observed, the budget constitutes the fiscal template that molds the profile of the department's programmatic activities.[7] He goes on to say, quite correctly, that budgetary history is by far the most important element in budget formulation.[8] In other words, the most important variable that determines the size of this year's budget is last year's budget.[9] Consequently, what one observes is that the amount expended in any one program does not vary by more than zero to five percent in any two successive years.[10] This means, then, that the size and variety of departmental programs, in actual dollars, are remarkably stable from year to year, given normal economic periods.[11]

The advocates of zero-based budgeting have more influence on political leaders during election campaigns than after. This is because zero-based budgeting can only rarely be applied to complex budgeting systems that ultimately facilitate the financing of high-value human programs.

The city's fiscal year runs from July 1 to June 30, and budget preparation usually commences in September, nine months before the new fiscal year. Within the Department of Health, the budget is formulated within numerous administrative and programmatic loci under the direction of the Deputy Commissioner for Administrative Services or the individual with similar authorities. Budget examiners are generally assigned to specific departments on a continuous basis by the Office of Management and Budget. Their task is to assist in the budget formulation process and to oversee the budget during the fiscal year. It would be erroneous, however, to conclude that their relationship with the health department is not often adversarial. Unlike the directors of service programs, their goal is to reduce or limit expenditures and to shift funds from one department to another in response to the mayor's larger political and administrative goals. The department's goal is to preserve the integrity of its budget at a minimum and to expand it as much as possible. These differences bring departmental and budgetary staff into ongoing dialogue, frequent conflict, and agreement at regular intervals.

There is frequent turnover of budget examiners, and they are often reassigned to cover other departments. This means that health department staff must frequently brief new examiners who lack detailed knowledge of the goals and effects of public health programs. Health department staff must act as both advocates and educators for public health programs as far as budget examiners are concerned. Because the performance of budget examiners is frequently measured by their superiors in terms of financial savings, their goal is to reduce funding. This, coupled with weak health department advocacy, can result in budget examiners deciding fiscal policy for the department.

Once Department of Health staff and the Office of Management and Budget agree on the budget, it is then put into final form, approved by the mayor, and submitted to the Finance Committee of the City Council and to the Board of Estimate. Public hearings at which health department staff and the Commissioner of Health testify and answer inquiries are held before both bodies. Frequently, members of the City Council and the Board of Estimate, being elected officials, try to use such hearings to political advantage. They often attempt to demonstrate their own fiscal responsibility by questioning various line items in the budget, picked out by their aides because they make good copy in the next day's press. Admixed with lines of inquiry having political motives are those based on sincere objective concern. Most health department officials who appear before these groups realize that excoriating interrogations are not aimed at them personally, but are usually undertaken in the political interests of the questioners. The staff work performed for these various officials is quite uneven in quality, and this is much in evidence at hearings.

Although the Board of Estimate has eight members, the comptroller, mayor, city council president and the five borough presidents, the votes are cast differently. The mayor, comptroller and city council president each have two votes, while the borough presidents have one. This means that the citywide officials can outvote the borough presidents. However, since 1975, when the new charter went into effect, the mayor is prohibited from voting on his budget. This prohibition does not extend to the other activities of the Board of Estimate, which involve public contracts and real estate transactions.

In recent years, hearings before the City Council and the Board of Estimate have produced only minor modifications in the Department of Health's budget. At certain times, members of these bodies have been extremely supportive of specific departmental programs and have assisted in raising the level of city funding for them.

COMPOSITION OF THE BUDGET

Monies within the Department of Health budget fall into three broad categories: city tax levy, state, and federal funds. It is the city tax levy which receives the major focus of attention by the Office of Management and Budget because these are monies that must be provided from city revenues. New York State has matched the city's public health expenditure at an average of fifty percent for many years. And the Department of Health has received sizeable sums in federal grants. This matching has served as a deterrent to the city's cutting back of funding because each reduction results in an equal loss of state monies. However, in recent years the state has lowered the level of its matching so that in 1981 to 1982 it was on the order of only 42 percent.

During the city's fiscal crisis, a number of federally funded programs were transferred out of the department's budget to the Medical and Health Research Association (see Chapter 5). This was done to bypass the unreasonable spending and hiring restrictions that the city temporarily imposed on all monies, and to benefit from MHRA's considerably lower overhead charges. Consequently, these monies do not appear in the department's regular budget.

In 1981, the Department of Health's expense budget was $111.4 million. Of this amount, $67.7 million was city tax levy, $31.3 million state matching monies and $12.4 million federal grant funds. Most of the budget went for personnel services, which amounted to $68.8 million. Other than personnel services amounted to $42.6 million. The personnel budget supported 3,435 full-time individuals and 600 part-time ones. The significant points in this budget were that state matching had dropped by 8 percent from the late 1970s and that although the city had made up for the loss with tax levy, the eroding effect of 12 percent annual inflation had dramatically reduced the effectiveness of the department's budget, and the budget continued to dwindle.

Since the early 1970s, the department has not had a capital budget. And with the advent of the fiscal crisis any hope of having one in the near future disappeared.

BUDGET REVIEWS

The department's budget is regularly subjected to both internal and external reviews. The latter are conducted by the comptroller, the Office of Management and Budget, the City Council, the Board of Estimate, and by funding agencies of the State of New York. Bellin points out that comprehensive annual budget reviews are simply not possible because they would require monies and staff few governments possess.[12] Consequently, many such reviews are superficial. On the average, Department of Health programs and their budgets received in-depth review every five years. However, since the 1975 fiscal crisis, the frequency of such reviews has been increased. Indeed, from 1975 on, departmental executives and managers spent most of their time dealing with budget and fiscal matters almost to the exclusion of all else. Programs were thus subjected to intense and ongoing scrutiny.

Chapter 11

THE DECISION-MAKING PROCESS

The decision-making process and policy formulation in the New York City Department of Health are affected by a number of variables. These include both internal and external checks and balances on authority and power, budgetary forces, competition among professional staff, the influx of new personnel, the appearance of new technologies, vogues, and the influence of pressure groups.

CHECKS AND BALANCES

The formal external checks and balances upon the department derive from the city's charter. It defines the department's authorities, powers, and areas of concern. In addition, court decisions and legislation at the state and local level, including that of the board of health, further define the department's role with regard to specific issues and programs. The department's regulatory and standard-setting activities are also checked by federal laws and regulations governing similar areas.

Because the Commissioner of Health is a member of the executive branch of municipal government, he must act within the broad policy directions set forth by the mayor. This serves as a check upon the department's activities, except when commissioners act differently because of a conflict with professional standards.

Public opinion and public sentiment also influence the policies of the department and play a role in the formulation of policy. In so doing, they act as a check upon the department's powers and activities.

BUDGETARY FORCES

The decision-making process is strongly influenced by budgetary forces. The generous funding of an area of public health concern by federal, state, or local sources almost automatically produces public health programs. For example, little was done about the mounting heroin addiction problem in New York City until large federal and state funds were made available to the Department of Health. These resulted in the decision to establish a network of methadone maintenance programs in the city.

Health department programs are regularly reviewed, although the periodicity of reviews is variable. During a period of fiscal stringency, the chances of individual programmatic review increase. And during exceptionally difficult fiscal times, such as those that occurred in 1975 and 1976, program directors must make herculean efforts to preserve their programs by justifying them to the Office of Management and Budget and the mayor. But even such justifications are sometimes inadequate.

For example, in 1975 the department expanded its capacity to accumulate data on window falls by children in the city.[1] Because of the high mortality associated with falls, the department launched an intervention program that consisted of purchasing window guards and distributing them in an experimental poverty area and in a control area. In the former, guards were distributed whether or not families requested them, and in the latter, only if they requested them. An educational program was instituted in the poverty area but not in the control one. At the end of one year, the project was evaluated and the results demonstrated a dramatic decline in the incidence of window falls among children in the experimental poverty area as compared to the control area.[2]

During the fiscal crisis, the Office of Management and Budget eliminated what had been a growing city allocation for this program despite the objections of the health department. Dr. Lowell E. Bellin, then Commissioner of Health, concluded that: (1) the window guard program was of vital importance and had to be expanded; (2) that someone other than the city had to finance the program, and it could not be the poor because they could not pay; (3) that landlords would have to pay the costs, there already being adequate precedents for their paying for other safety features such as electric outlets and concealed wiring; (4) that the City Council would never pass such a law;

and (5) that the Board of Health might pass it if the action were perceived as one involving the public health.[3]

At Bellin's request, the Board of Health considered the issue carefully and then promulgated a health code regulation (Section 131.15) that requires landlords of buildings with three or more families to furnish window guards, except on windows providing access to fire escapes, in apartments where children ten years of age and younger reside. Predictably, a realtor group brought suit in the courts, arguing that the Board of Health had exceeded its legal authority in passing a regulation that dealt with safety rather than public health. The Board of Health's counsel persuasively argued that safety was a subset of public health, and the court ruled in the board's favor.[4]

During the time that the suit was in progress, the health department was subjected to substantial political pressures generated by both realtors and some elected political officials.[5] The department and the board stood firm on their position, even though this brought them into direct conflict with a powerful economic interest group and powerful officials.

COMPETITION AMONG PROFESSIONAL STAFF

A health commissioner of New York City has never been in a position in recent years to consistently impose his will on the hierarchical levels below him. Rather, he or she is in a constant state of negotiation with subordinates. In order to retain the skills and loyalty of highly desirable staff, a commissioner must be responsive to their interests. These interests include not only working conditions, a fair share of the budget and salaries, but also the public health objectives they champion. Understandably, professionals compete for position in a hierarchical structure that is pyramidal. As Bellin notes, in this competitive process professionals consciously identify themselves as champions of specific policies and programs that advance their objectives.[6] In effect, these policies and programs act as surrogates for the advocating professionals. It is through them that professionals advance their own careers. To be successful, professionals must also see to it that their programs succeed. Thus, they enhance productivity, efficiency, and effectiveness, modify the program as needed, and advocate it to the point of personifying it.

The decision-making process is strongly affected by the dynamics of professional competition. In fact, the process often emerges out of this competition. And the health commissioner not infrequently finds himself in the position of being a ratifier and reviewer of decisions made by his subordinates in which their competitive interests play a significant role.

THE INFLUX OF NEW PROFESSIONALS

New professionals predictably try to put their imprint on the functions and activities that come under their supervision. They usually undertake a fresh and in-depth look at programs and sometimes take bold initiatives. There may not be much staying power in these actions, as sooner or later the new professional absorbs much of the old system as it does him. He eventually becomes an accepted part of the bureaucracy. But while the newness lasts, these professionals can bring about major structural and functional changes.

NEW TECHNOLOGY

Technological advances make possible public health programs that otherwise would not exist. As Bellin cogently observes, technology renders certain programs possible, but it does not alone guarantee that such programs will be implemented.[7] Technological advances often have a profound effect on current programs. They may negate the need for existing procedures and certain categories of jobs in addition to making possible greatly expanded public services. Consequently, while greeted with support by potential beneficiaries, they are often viewed as undesirable by those whose jobs may be altered by them.

VOGUES

Trends are frequently set in the field of public health by leading professionals, health departments, and learned consensus. These vogues may or may not last, depending on empirical observations of their value. For example, the annual physical examination, once viewed as an effective tool of preventive medicine, has now been shown by many to be of limited value. Other vogues last for even shorter periods of time. They are initiated after convincing proof is produced by someone or some group, the proof in retrospect often not so convincing, and quickly espoused by leading authorities. Frequently, a momentum that obscures its weaknesses is generated behind a vogue. And it is only after some time has passed and the vogue has lost its glamour that probing doubts are raised. It is often difficult for public health department) to call for careful and measured scrutiny of these proposals, given their popular and political support.

Other vogues have validity and longer staying power, such as the lead poisoning control program initiated by the New York City Department of Health in the early 1970s.[8] The department had had a rather casual policy about lead poisoning until Chicago's health department undertook wide-scale screening and found that a high percentage of children in poverty areas had abnormally high blood lead levels.[9] In 1969, it was estimated that there were some 121,000 children between the ages of one and six living in New York City in housing where there was a likelihood of their being exposed to lead-based paint.[10] Yet no attempt was made to address this problem until it had been spotlighted in other localities and until lead poisoning advocates and journalists put pressure on the department to do something about the problem.

One of the interventions designed was apartment repair, which cost approximately $1,500 per unit. Eventually, a careful program evaluation found that apartment repair did not affect the recidivism rate. Yet it was a loudly demanded service because program beneficiaries perceived it as having great value. Thus, it was retained despite its questionable value.

PRESSURE GROUPS

Pressure groups have historically played a significant role in the decision-making processes of the health department. New York City's pressure group system is complex and has undergone considerable change in the past several years, especially in the field of health. In recent decades, the major political parties have not functioned as pressure groups on the Department of Health. This is due in part to the fact that the city is so dominated by the Democratic party, which is composed of heterogeneous ethnic and religious affiliations. Elected officials who bring pressure to bear on the Department of Health do so not because of party affiliation but because of a need to be responsive to the demands of heterogeneous constituencies. Most of the contact between the department and various elected officials such as councilmen, state senators, state assemblymen, borough presidents, and congressmen is rather benign. The latter frequently write letters advocating a decision favorable to constituents but have no serious intention of influencing the decision. The purpose is merely to demonstrate a responsiveness to their constituents' voiced demands. On matters of greater import, and such may occur only a few times a year as far as they are concerned, they first attempt to influence through the mayor's office and, if unsuccessful, will deal directly with the department.

Overall, pressures from elected officials are miniscule when compared to those generated by other segments of the pressure group system. Bornfriend has cogently observed that there are two broad categories of groups within this system.[11] The first consists of "established" groups and the second of "newcomers." The established groups consist of a number of civic, religious, philanthropic, professional, labor, and business organizations. In health, the New York Academy of Medicine and the county medical societies were once powerful professional pressure groups. But in the past two decades, they have gradually reduced their pressure group roles. Other established groups, such as the City Club and the Citizen's Committee for Children, have, however, increased theirs.

As Bornfriend points out, organizations such as those just mentioned have remained relatively stable in terms of type of membership and areas of concern. There is great similarity in the tactics they use to influence decisions, shaped in large measure by years of experience and sophistication in the use of the political process. The established groups prefer to exert their influence by appearing at public hearings, meeting with elected and appointed office holders, having members serve on boards and committees, and exerting influence on mayors concerning the appointment of health officials.

Bornfriend underscores a number of other structural and functional characteristics of established groups.[12] As a rule, they remain viable in the political process even if they consistently fail to achieve their goals. Their members, who are professionals, do not pay dues, with the expectation of the leadership achieving these goals. They do so for professional recognition, status, and access to certain services such as symposia, lectures, and journals that provide them with both technical and practical information. Most members of such groups have no desire to be activists in the political process and are usually either unaware or disinterested in the executives' activities in this area.

On the balance sheet, the activities of established medical societies have exerted a positive influence on public health in the city. They have given their support to commissioners of health on decisions which, while in the best interests of the public, have often encountered serious opposition from small groups of vocal opponents. And over the years they have won the respect of political leaders of all persuasions through their careful and studied approaches to issues and the soundness of their recommendations.

The second large segment of the pressure group system consists of the "newcomers" as Bornfriend defines them.[13] This category includes an enormous number of groups formed around the issues of poverty, welfare, employment, neighborhoods, and race. Most are composed of Blacks and Puerto Ricans. While the established groups consider relationships with government and involvement in the political process as only one of their many activities, the newcomers direct all of their energies at government because, as they see it, their demands can only be met in the public sector.[14] While the membership of the New York Academy of Medicine judges the performance of its leadership on the basis of the quality of symposia, lectures, newsletters, and a scientific journal, a neighborhood poverty group's leadership provides no services. Their effectiveness, therefore, hinges on their success in winning objectives for their constituents. Failure to do so places them in jeopardy within the organization. Thus, the internal pressures on the leaders of newcomer groups to achieve political goals are far greater than those on established group leaders.

The leadership of the newcomer groups must resort to highly visible high pressure tactics such as demonstrations, sit-ins, strikes, holding officials captive, and destroying property in order to preserve their own internal group position and convince their constituents of their effectiveness as leaders. While they may not deliver on the goal, they almost never fail to deliver on process. It is this often violent process that attracts news media coverage that gives status to the newcomer group and enhances its leadership. Newcomer groups in the health field, as do others in other fields, often take non-negotiable positions, and their proven ability to quickly mobilize sympathizers willing to support these positions only serves to harden them all the more.

As the city's financial resources dwindled during the early 1970s and the fiscal crisis was perceived by even the newcomers as real and not fabricated, changes in tactics were discernable. Violent protests by the workers of one hospital threatened by closure no longer won sympathy among those at other hospitals. The exchange of support once so freely given dwindled in the shadow of the reality that there were not enough resources to go around. By the late 1970s many of the newcomer groups had matured enough to adopt the strategies of their older established cousins. News coverage was no longer a sure asset to their causes. Backlash by other groups, both established and newcomer, grew. Although the glare of protest is still sought by some, it is no longer the sure ticket to the fulfillment of expectations. The expansion of newcomer "service demanders" and the dwindling of the resources of "service providers" finally struck home as a harsh reality of the city's present life.

HOW DECISIONS ARE MADE

Most public health policy decisions do not represent massive quantum leaps in any direction. Seasoned health commissioners in New York City have tended to be cautious, taking undramatic steps, except in extraordinary circumstances. Wise health commissioners have usually used new technologies in demonstration projects prior to employing them in mass programs. They have known of colleagues or have heard of colleagues who have paid dearly for bold steps into the unknown. Courage tempered by prudence is not to be scorned.[15]

Data are important in the decision making process, but they represent, as Bellin notes, but a single category of interdependent variables that contribute to making a public decision. He goes on to say that data are useful in detecting longitudinal trends, and in formulating rough ideas about the content, magnitude and complexity of a problem.[16] But administrative decisions within the Department of Health have characteristically been based on approximation and improvisation rather than precision and influenced by all or some of the factors discussed above.[17]

Bellin has provided a masterly analysis of how some of these variables inter-relate. As he shows, the initiative for a policy or program may begin either inside or outside the Department of Health. New programs need both inside and outside support if they are to be transformed from conception to promulgation.[18] Eventually, new programs become absorbed and functionally integrated into the general activities of the department. Subordinate staff are the constituencies of superordinates. And superordinates are in a state of constant negotiation with subordinates. If the superordinate does not deliver with reasonable frequency on behalf of the subordinates' interests, he risks losing their loyalty and support.[19] Such interests include not merely salaries, fringe benefits, working conditions and promotions, but also professional gratifications as well. These interests, Bellin points out, also include the public health objectives that these constituents champion.

The impetus for making decisions usually comes from below the level of the top executives in the department who are primarily reviewers and ratifiers. True, commissioners and their deputies sometimes initiate the process, but this is infrequent when compared to its frequency at lower levels.

Interlocking with the professional subordinates within the department are new technologies, vogues, budgetary forces and extra-departmental constituencies and pressure groups. Outside constituencies and pressure groups sometimes form alliances with pertinent people on the health department staff to foster the advancement of specific programs. And professional staff often solicit informal support from such groups in order to advance programs of mutual interest.

As in any democratic institution, decisions are made through processes affected by numerous variables. Only rarely does the commissioner alone or working with a few deputies make a decision or formulate a new policy. As Bellin notes, public health administrators are more comfortable with undramatic incrementalism, with reviewing and ratifying decisions made by subordinates, weighing in such variables as new technologies, professional competition, public health need and constraints imposed by the sociopolitical environment and the budget.[20]

Chapter 12

INTERFACING WITH
THE STATE GOVERNMENT

The New York City Department of Health interfaces with a number of federal, state, and local governmental agencies. However, its most important relationship has been with the New York State Department of Health and the temporary health bureaucracies created by various governors. The size and quality of the city health department overshadowed the state health department for many decades. This derived from the fact that the former had to respond to the ever-growing problems of a large and heterogeneous urban population. Consequently, it was on the cutting edge of public health progress and attracted large numbers of talented public health professionals. The state health department, on the other hand, was concerned for many years with a primarily small, stable, rural population. This, coupled with the existence of many county health departments, let to an evaluation of the state health department as a second best organization with limited depth of interest. Few would attempt to argue the learned concensus that the state's department was, in reality, a very poor relation of the city's department. As the city's department scored one success after another and gradually became a model for health departments all over the country, the state's department simply rocked along. True, the state's department did occasionally benefit from the leadership of outstanding public health professionals. But in the main it held second place to the city's department.

This situation began to change in the mid-1960s, with the expansion of regulatory functions related to government supported medical care such as Medicaid. Prior to that time, governors had not been anxious for their health departments to assume service responsibilities in the city, as these carried unwanted political liabilities. Standard setting and regulation, however, were, in a political sense, less hazardous. Thus, as their importance grew, the state health department increasingly assumed these responsibilities. Some were delegated to the city health department, which was held accountable to the state. This placed the two departments in a working relationship that was closer than what had existed before. At the same time, the city's long-standing independence from the state and the decentralization of local powers that had characterized government in the state for many decades was drawing to an end. There was a palpable shift toward centralization at the state level and a marked erosion of the once sacred political philosophy of "home rule." With the advent of the fiscal crisis in 1975, these trends accelerated because the state had to move aggressively into city affairs in order to prevent certain bankruptcy.

During the late 1960s and early 1970s the state assumed a number of inspectional functions from the city health department over the strong objections of several city health commissioners. While some of these functions were transferred to the state health department, others went to other state agencies such as the Department of Agriculture and Markets. These transfers had always been championed by regulated industries and businesses because the longer arm of the state has usually been less efficient at enforcement than the city health department. The state health department's choices were characterized by the fact that they were usually nonservice functions devoid of pressure group interest and political jeopardy.

In addition, state monitoring of the city health department's functions intensified because the state provided matching funds for many programs and also because the city was the state's delegate with regard to these programs. Toward the mid-1970s, prior to the advent of the fiscal crisis, all of these dynamics frequently led to a tense and acrimonious relationship betwee the two health departments. The aim of state health department officials was to acquire key public health functions in the city. These functions were eventually sufficiently numerous and significant to warrant the opening of a regional office in the city. City health department officials understandably resisted these attempts and saw their department reduced to that of a residuary with a potpourri of functions unwanted by the state.

The state picked and chose the functions it wanted, leaving the city department with the bulk of undesired personal services and regulatory and inspectional functions that could not yet be absorbed. There was unanimity of opinion among both city public health officials and others that quality generally suffered whenever the state took over a function. This assessment, although suspect coming from city officials, was verified by the fact that the state frequently lacked both the necessary resources and the political will to carry out these functions. Many city public health officials argued that state takeover was simply a convenient means of suspending a program by rendering it inactive. They pointed out that when the city department ran the quality assurance component of the Medicaid program, providers were regularly cited for fraud, overutilization and poor-quality care. Yet when the state successfully wrested the program from the city health department after a court battle, judging from the state's enforcement record, an epidemic of honesty broke out among providers.

It is tempting to assess the state-city conflict over public health services as merely a power struggle between two competing bureaucracies. But such a reductionist approach falls far from the mark because the conflict stemmed from divergent philosophies of government. It is easier still to view objecting city public health officials as waging battle merely to preserve power and status. This, too, is simplistic because it ignores the philosophical commitment of these individuals to an independent health department and their professional and emotional links to a long tradition of excellence. This, after all, was the department of John Rice, Ernest Stebbins, Harry Mustard, Leona Baumgartner, George James, Mary McLaughlin, and Lowell Bellin. The roots of the conflict lay not in bureaucratic struggle or fears of loss of power, but in divergent philosophies of what was best for the public health and how best to achieve it. The state's philosophy was based on the concept of centralization, with the establishment of regional centers under state control. Crucial to the city health department's philosophy was local independence based on the principle of home rule. And behind it stood a long record of achievement to prove that it had worked, and worked well. The low professional opinion of the state health department held by city public health officials, and the tinge of envy with which the former viewed the city health department, were but nonessential additives to the ongoing conflict.

The fiscal crisis of 1975 intensified the conflict because state officials had a freer hand to move into the city's affairs, the mayor and his administration were in desperate fiscal straits and cooperative to a degree heretofore unknown, and city public health officials were determined to preserve what they believed to be the best local health department in the United States. The conflict erupted into a major confrontation in early 1977 when the state made a frontal assault against the city health department in the from of a proposal to establish the temporary position of "health czar." This proposal, had it been carried through to fruition, might have resulted in the dismantling of the New York City Department of Health. While the position ostensibly proposed to deal with hospital problems, the health czar was to have full authority over the city's health commissioner and, in turn, report to both the governor's special advisor for health and the city's first deputy mayor. Disregarding for the moment the structural deficiencies of such an arrangement, it is worth noting that the city health department had no hospital responsibilities or involvement per se in hospitals and, consequently, need not have been incorporated into such a scheme. It was clear that the state's intentions extended beyond hospital issues.

The health czar proposal provides an excellent case study not only of city-state relations, but also of conflict between a health commissioner and a mayor. For in this case the mayor was willing to endorse the proposal in order to solicit gubernatorial support in an upcoming mayoral election. Thus, the health department found itself pitted against both the mayor and those state officials who favored the proposal. Interestingly, the state health department, long at the interface of conflict with the city health deparment, was not involved in what turned out to be a crisis of major proportions for the latter.

BACKGROUND TO THE HEALTH CZAR PROPOSAL

The city's fiscal crisis essentially constituted the broad canvas out of which the health czar proposal emerged (see Chapters 1 and 5). In September 1975, Governor Hugh Carey effectively removed financial management of the city's affairs from Mayor Abraham Beame.[1] He did so by calling a special session of the state legislature and obtaining its approval for the creation of the Emergency Financial Control Board (EFCB) on which the state had a voting majority.[2]

The board was given broad powers, including the approval of most city contracts and disbursement authority over all revenues received by the city or by so-called public benefit corporations and agencies such as the Transit Authority, the Board of Education, and the Health and Hospitals Corporation (HHC). All monies collected by these organizations were deposited with the EFCB and could only be disbursed after it had approved spending plans. In addition, a special deputy state comptroller was appointed to audit the city's books and supervise financial reporting.[3] The results of establishing these safeguards were that the banks agreed to roll over notes and the pension funds agreed to buy bonds issued by the Municipal Assistance Corporation (MAC). Also, the state's own fiscal situation was safeguarded.

Clearly, then, the state, with a voting majority on the EFCB, was effectively in charge of the city's fiscal affairs. And whoever holds the purse strings has the determining voice in policy decisions. By the end of 1976, the focus of the EFCB was sharpened on the HHC because financial plans submitted by the latter had been deemed unacceptable. As 1977 dawned, the HHC projected a two-year deficit of $140 million, something unacceptable to the EFCB and those who were financing the city through its fiscal crisis.[4] On January 12 1977, the board of the HHC approved a two-year plan aimed at easing this projected deficit.[5] This plan had been drawn up under the direction of both the HHC and the city's Office of Management and Budget. The essential elements of the plan included revenue producing measures, such as accelerated collections and higher rates from third-party payers like Medicaid and Blue Cross, and increased city and state funding. The plan included some contingencies, such as hospital closures and the consolidation of services at four other hospitals, which could have led to a loss of 1,143 jobs.[6] The two hospitals that would have been closed were Sydenham in Harlem, a small acute care facility, and Bird S. Coler on Roosevelt Island, a chronic disease hospital. Funding reductions would have affected Elmhurst Hospital and the Queens Hospital Center.[7] Employee and community opposition to all of these proposed attrition measures was strong and vocal. In fact, the HHC board meeting that approved this plan met in the auditorium of Pace University so as to accommodate the large crowd of speakers and protestors. It was clear that there was no unity among diverse employee and community groups, each aware that the preservation of their institutions could only be had at the expense of someone else's.

The political pressures generated by potentially affected workers and communities was enormous. And later in the day, after the HHC Board had approved the plan, Harlem leaders met with Mayor Beame to convey the community's anger and disgust at the threatened closing of Sydenham.[8] The mayor was up for reelection later in the year and therefore unlikely to support hospital closures.[9]

It was obvious to most that the plan, heavily dependent as it was on revenue enhancement measures and additional state and city funding, was an uncertain formula for dealing with HHC's deficits. The following week the EFCB rejected it. The executive director of the EFCB had previously been critical of the then current management of the HHC and the EFCB, in addition to rejecting the HHC financial plan expressed lack of confidence in the current HHC management to produce an acceptable money saving plan.[10] Because of the enormity of the HHC operating budget, the EFCB, concerned as it was with the city's financial recovery, feared that failure to produce an acceptable plan would jeopardize its broader efforts. This point of view was expressed to the mayor and to members of the HHC board. It carried enormous weight because the EFCB had a great deal of control over the city's affairs, and direct control over HHC's spending. It was this series of events which led to the removal of the HHC president by the HHC board on January 26, 1977.

The EFCB made clear its lack of confidence in the president of the HHC and communicated this to the mayor.[11] Mayor Beame then attempted, unsuccessfully, to get the president to resign. The president of the HHC, Dr. John Holloman, was a prominent black physician widely respected as a humane and compassionate doctor. But many on the board of the HHC as well as those on the EFCB had serious doubts that he could successfully lead the corporation out of its financial difficulties. Consequently, the board of the HHC met on January 26, 1977, and after seven hours of deliberation voted by nine to seven to remove him as president 12-14. Significantly, District Council 37, the union that represented the corporation's 18,000 employees, most of whom were minorities, did not support him.[15] In fact, Victor Gotbaum, the head of the union, publicly called Holloman incompetent.[16]

District Council 37 had a larger concern, its sinking of substantial amounts of its pension funds into city bonds as part of the fiscal recovery program. Thus, it was not surprising that the union that might otherwise have supported Holloman gave its tacit approval to his removal.[17] Holloman was supported by Percy Sutton, the black borough president of Manhattan, who announced his candidacy in the upcoming mayoralty race the same day Holloman was removed, and by a small, vocal, heterogeneous group of people.[18]

Dr. Holloman remained on as president of the corporation until April 20, 1977. However, during that time the mayor moved to tighten his authority over the corporation's affairs. He did this both in the hopes of bringing about needed managerial changes and to demonstrate a resolve to the EFCB that he favored this kind of tighter control. In addition, it was the concensus opinion of the EFCB and both state and city governments that the HHC budget deficits could not be eliminated without service reductions and even hospital closures.[19] And this could not be achieved without behind the scenes mayoral control of the HHC, which at that time really meant state control.

While these attempts were underway, the mayor launched an informal search for a replacement for Dr. Holloman. The foremost candidate was Deputy Schools Chancellor Bernard R. Gifford, a highly respected black administrator, who later made an unsuccessful bid for a congressional seat in Brooklyn.[20,21] However, he eventually withdrew interest in the HHC presidency.[20]

Meanwhile, Governor Carey and his special assistant for health affairs, Dr. Kevin M. Cahill, put forth a major reorganization of the state's health bureaucracy on February 17, 1977. This reorganization, which was later put into effect, included the creation of a new Office of Health Systems Management within the state health department.[22] Eventually, this office came to have gubernatorial cabinet status, although legally it was still a part of the health department. Its principal role was to set rates and standards for hospitals, nursing homes, and clinics. These key functions had previously been under the direct control of the state health commissioner. Consequently, the state health department lost a sizeable portion of its functions. These structural changes were said to be in the interests of controlling the state's escalating health care costs.

These organizational changes in the state's health buraucracy were announced as part of the governor's State of the Health message to the legislature. In it he also called for centralization of the certificate of need process under Dr. Cahill, also chairman of the State Health Planning Commission. As one journalist observed, "...Dr. Kevin Cahill, Governor Hugh Carey's $1 a year health adviser and top personal adviser would get new powers under the governor's plan for reorganizing the state's health bureaucracy...Dr. Cahill, a specialist in tropical diseases who did most of the work on Carey's second special message on health will chair new committees, prepare health care systems master plans and become a virtual czar in controlling construction of virtually all new health and mental health facilities...''[23]

In sum, the state had dramatically moved in the direction of centralization of control over health matters under a staff person who was simultaneously personal physician, chief health adviser, and adviser to the governor on other matters as well.[14,25] Part of this plan, as laid out in the governor's February 17, 1977 State of the Health message, included the creation of a health czar jointly appointed by the governor and the mayor, who would report to both the city's first deputy mayor and to Dr. Cahill. This proposal was predictably lauded in an editorial by the *New York Daily News* whose editor was both a friend and supporter of the governor.[26] And it was fully supported by the EFCB, a gubernatorial creation.[27] Other newspapers supported the idea as well, arguing that a unified command could lead to a resolution of the city's hospital problems.[28] These arguments had great appeal for a public wearied by protracted stalemates of state and city attempts to deal with the ever-rising deficits of the HHC and spiraling health care costs. They ignored, however, the great hidden agenda of the health czar proposal: to create a position seemingly vested with sweeping powers to make such unpalatable decisions as closing hospitals, and yet one several steps removed from a governor whose appointed officials already had such powers. Health czardom was really a means of achieving these unpopular ends, while at the same time providing the governor with protective cover from their political consequences.

THE FIRST PROPOSAL

The first formal notice of the governor's proposal for a health czar was given to me as health commissioner at a city hall meeting on Monday, February 21, 1977. The meeting was chaired by John Zuccotti, then Mayor Beame's first deputy mayor. Zuccotti, a highly respected administrator and manager and former head of the city's Planning Commission, took a special interest in health affairs. He was held in very high esteem by myself and the executives and managers of the health department. Zuccotti possessed an excellent working knowledge of the city's health care system and problems. Also in attendance were Donald Kummerfeld, then Director of the city's Office Of Management and Budget, who had major responsibilities in the HHC, and his assistants. Zuccotti's principal assistant was also there.

Zuccotti related that the health czar would essentially become a deputy commissioner of health for New York City affairs in the state health department, chairman of the Inter-Agency Health Council, a member of the executive committee of the Health Systems Agency, principal health adviser to the mayor, and the immediate superior to the health commissioner of New York City.[29] The stated intent of the governor's health czar proposal was to address urgent problems in the health care delivery system, especially those in hospitals.

The objections that I raised about this proposal at this meeting centered upon two broad areas, its complex structure, in which the city health commissioner would report to two individuals, and its inclusion of the city's public health department in a new bureaucracy established to handle hospital problems. A fuller understanding of these objections requires some knowledge of the city's health bureaucracy at the time. The health commissioner was then the mayor's principal health advisor and chairman of the Inter-Agency Health Council, a grouping of the commissioners of health, mental health, addiction services, human resources, and the head of the HHC. The council rarely met and at the time its role was poorly defined. In addition, the health commissioner was the Health Services Administrator, a title without much functional significance since the Health Services Administration had been disbanded. However, the Health Services Administrator was by law chairman of the HHC board. Thus, the health commissioner was both chairman and a member of the board, with two votes. The health commissioner was also chairman of the executive committee of the Health Systems Agency. Although the health commissioner played a key role in the HHC, the health department did not.

Zuccotti was receptive to these objections and said he would raise them with Cahill later in the week when they met to negotiate the proposal. Meanwhile, a full text of the proposal was given to the Department of Health.

THE STATE'S PROPOSAL

The state's proposal called for the creation of a Director and Coordinator of Health for New York City. This proposal, as presented to the health department, read as follows:

> The director will be jointly appointed by the governor and the mayor. This shall be a temporary position through June 30, 1978. This position is required because of the obvious need to address urgent problems in the health care delivery system that are now under state, city and federal jurisdiction.
>
> In order to accomplish the charges listed below the director shall serve as the principal health advisor to the mayor and shall have vested in him all the necessary responsibilities by the state in order to fulfill his task. He shall report directly to the assistant to the governor for health affairs (Kevin M. Cahill) and the first deputy mayor (John Zuccotti).
>
> In the city, the New York City Commissioner of Health shall report to director with respect to the responsibilities listed below. Furthermore he will chair the Inter-Agency Health Council (consisting of the Commissioner of Health, Mental Health, Addiction Services, and Social Services, the President of the Health and Hospital Corporation, and the Director of Management and Budget). The executive director of the HSA will be asked to be represented on the Inter-Agency Health Council.
>
> He shall serve in lieu of the first deputy mayor as his permanent alternate on the board and executive committee of the Health Systems Agency for New York City. The director shall review and approve the budget and plans (as well as the location, type, service, and facilities) of the NYC Health and Hospitals Corporation before submission by the city to the EFCB.
>
> The state shall also appoint the director to serve as deputy director of the State Health Planning Commission and delegate him the responsibilities and functions of that commission in New York City.

GOALS AND RESPONSIBILITIES

Specifically the Director will:

1. Develop, identify, and institute policies to:
   a. Consolidate the institutional system of health care delivery by eliminating un-needed facilities and un-used capacity.

This shall apply to the municipal, voluntary and proprietary hospital systems as well as the long-term care facilities.

b. Improve the efficiency of the health care delivery system by eliminating duplicative services, and by encouraging the development of ambulatory services and other alternate and more cost-effective forms of care.

c. Establish a regional system of health care so that access to the reduced system is guaranteed to those in need of medical care.

2. Serve as the city's and state's liaison with the federal government on all policy matters relating to the reimbursement of health care services in the city of New York.

3. Review and comment on all systems used for regulating and financing health care in New York City to ensure that these are consistent with a consolidated system able to provide necessary health care.

4. Reshape existing regulatory programs to clearly delineate responsibility, reduce administrative costs, and ensure an effective review of providers to protect the interests of the state city and the recipients of care.

STAFFING AND OFFICES

The director and his staff shall receive joint support from the city and state. It is estimated that a staff of 10-15 professional level people will be required some of which can be transferred from existing lines on the city and state level.

The director as the chief health advisor to the mayor shall have his office space similar to those assigned to deputy mayors.

REACTION OF THE NEW YORK DEPARTMENT OF HEALTH

On Tuesday, February 22, 1977, I called a meeting of all the deputy and associate commissioners of the Department of Health. They were given detailed information about the health czar proposal. A number argued that if the proposal went through, the city health department would become an appendage of the governor's office. Resources would be diverted from it to the office of the health czar and the health commissioner's position denigrated. The structure of the office, consisting as it did of an individual responsible to both a first deputy mayor (a line position) and the governor's special assistant for health affairs (a staff position), defied organizational wisdom. Most thought it unworkable.

Some cogently pointed out that since the health czar was being appointed to manage hospital problems, there was then no need to include the city health department. And all present saw an ethical and legal problem for the health commissioner in his role as the HHC board chairman. Because the health czar would be the health commissioner's immediate superior, he would be in a position to direct the health commissioner in his capacity as chairman of the HHC board. This would be in violation of state law, which holds that a member of a corporate board owes his loyalty to the corporation and cannot be influenced or directed by outside forces adverse to the interests of the corporation. Others raised the possibility that the health czar could use the health commissioner in his capacity as HHC board chairman as an agent to implement his plans, and that since these were likely to be unpopular he would bear the brunt of community and worker anger.

It was the consensus of the Department of Health's top staff that the health czar proposal was the most serious assault ever made on the department, and that if it were allowed to go through, it would result in serious damage to the department. No one objected to the governor's use of this new position to deal with the city's intractable hospital problems because all other efforts had so far failed. Thus, it was suggested that Zuccotti negotiate to change the health czar's role to that of a special adviser to the mayor for hospital affairs and not have the health commissioner report to the health czar. Clearly, the city had to offer something in return and it was suggested by my staff that I give the health czar the chairmanship of the HHC board. This would put him in a position to deal directly with the HHC and would remove both the Department of Health and its commissioner from the center of the hospital issue.

NEGOTIATIONS

During the next two weeks, Zuccotti tried unsuccessfully to negotiate a change to a hospital czar proposal with Cahill. The latter refused. In fact, Ronald Walter, Zuccotti's assistant who was involved in the negotiations, reported that Cahill was furious that I had tried to water down and alter the proposal.[30] He was also furious over the fact that on March 1, 1977, one of my deputy commissioners had made contact with a deputy commissioner in the state health department to discuss the health czar proposal. There was little enthusiasm for the proposal among many of the state's public health officials and mutual discussions of it seemed an alliance needed to defeat it.

Both Zuccotti and Mayor Beame were in a difficult negotiating position for three reasons. Because of the fiscal crisis, city officials were in a weak position. The state was, after all, firmly in control of the city's fiscal affairs. Second, Beame and Zuccotti were struggling to get the 1977-1978 city budget approved. And finally, Beame planned to run for reelection in the fall and both wanted and needed the governor's support. It had been rumored that if Beame did not run, then John Zuccotti would. Thus, he did not want to lock horns in a bitter struggle with the governor's closest adviser. Nonetheless he did try to negotiate, seeing the need to maintain an independent local health department and keep it separate from hospital issues. But he found that Cahill would negotiate nothing. The proposal had to be accepted as it was.

I had by this time reached the decision that it would be better to resign than to participate in a plan that posed ethical and legal problems and that would lead to the dismantling of the Department of Health.

On March 10, 1977, Zuccotti called me to an early morning meeting in the basement of the mayor's residence. He said that Cahill had refused to negotiate any changes in the proposal and that the mayor had finally decided to go along with it. He pointed out that if I continued my opposition, I would have to resign or be asked to resign. After consulting with a number of professionals both within the department and outside it, including some former city health commissioners, I decided to see the mayor myself. He and I had never discussed the proposal. In addition, I called an emergency meeting of the Board of Health in order to seek their support for the position I had taken on behalf of myself and the Department of Health. I saw the mayor at noon for only ten minutes as he had to leave for a meeting with Israel's prime minister. He raised two points. One was that the state health commissioner had already lost so many functions, and the other that the state wanted control over the

HHC.[31] When we met again at 2 P.M., I told him that simply because the state health commissioner had allowed an erosion of his department's functions was no reason for me to do the same. And if the state wanted control of the HHC they had only to appoint their health czar as board chairman and take the needed legal steps. The mayor indicated that he wanted to cooperate as much as he could with the governor, and I took this to mean that he saw that he had to in order to obtain the governor's support in the mayoralty race. I told the mayor that I could not accept the health czar proposal as it was structured and that if he wished, I would resign. He was genuinely shocked when I offered my resignation.

An hour later the Board of Health met. Only two of the four members attended, but the two who could not come had been contacted by phone and had given me their full support in opposing the health czar proposal as then structured. Throughout these efforts the Department of Health had received no constituency support for its position. Most tended to view our opposition in a reductionist manner, as based on fear of loss of prestige and power. And indeed, this was the view first expressed by the two members of the Board of Health who did attend the meeting. Members of the department's staff carefully listed the arguments against the proposal. True, the health commissioner would lose authority and power. But the department would also lose its independence, and its commissioner would be dragged into legal and ethical problems with regard to the HHC. What the state proposed was an administrative nightmare, a jointly apointed individual answering to two bosses, one city, and one state. The health commissioner, unlike any other commissioner in city government, would no longer report to the mayor but to the jointly appointd health czar. Finally, the two Board of Health members gave their assent to a resolution that read as follows:

WHEREAS the Department of Health of the City of New York has enjoyed a reputation as a center of excellence in the United States and throughout the world, and

WHEREAS the Department of Health suffered deprofessionalization of its staff during previous years, and

WHEREAS the reprofessionalization of the Department, under the leadership of the Mayor, has restored it once again to its former high level of excellence and effectiveness in serving the people of the City of New York,

NOW THEREFORE BE IT RESOLVED that in order for the Department of Health to continue to function at that high level of excellence in public health it is essential for the Commissioner of Health to continue to report directly to the Mayor of the City of New York and that he not be required formally to report to any Health Administrator who would be inserted between the Health Commissioner and the Mayor.

AND BE IT FURTHER RESOLVED that the Commissioner of Health shall not be placed in a position where he is compelled to suffer a conflict of interest in his positions as chairman of the Board of Health and Hospitals Corporation and as chairman of the executive committee of the Health Systems Agency.

Two days later, on March 12, 1977, the *New York Daily News*, whose editor Michael O'Neill was a friend of both the governor and Kevin Cahill, ran an editorial blasting me for my sustained opposition.[32] The editorial misrepresented the facts in that it claimed I was in favor of the proposal "on the record," but that I was privately using every bit of political muscle to abort the plan.[33]

On March 15, 1977, the same paper ran a guest editorial by Dr. Lowell E. Bellin, a former Commissioner of Health of the city and a former board chairman of the HHC.[34] In this editorial, Bellin eloquently argued that the health czar would simply be an official whipping boy for both the governor and the mayor. He went on to say that both the mayor and the governor were unwilling to surrender complete control of hospital closure to the other, that each wanted a substantial say but insubstantial onus, for saying it.[35] In this article, Bellin pointed out that the city health commissioner performed an important function as chairman of the Health Systems Agency executive committee. He also referred to the persuasive powers of the city health commissionership. Three days later, Cahill came back with a sharp letter of reply to Bellin in which he characterized the city health commissionership as an irrelevant position. And many in the health department thought it no coincidence that he then added the chairmanship of the Health Systems Agency's executive committee to the roles of the health czar. This placed the would-be health czar in another conflict because he would also be deputy director of the State Health Planning Commission, which reviewed decisions made by the executive committee of the New York City Health Systems Agency.

It is worth noting that Cahill, who in 1978 viewed the city health commissionership as an irrelevant position, in 1981 accepted appointment to the New York City Board of Health from Mayor Koch after he had had a falling out with Governor Carey.[36] Cahill resigned from his position as Carey's chief health advisor in December 1980. Later in 1981, Cahill agreed to screen candidates for Koch for a health commissionership that had been much reduced in prestige and scope in the three years since he had characterized it as irrelevant.

Mayor Beame and Zuccotti were in a bind. They did manage to change the wording of the proposal to read that the city health commissioner would report to the health czar only on hospitals, ambulatory care, and health care delivery matters. This excluded most health department functions. At this point, many who had once been enthusiastic about the proposal were now having second thoughts. And there were serious doubts that anyone could be found to fill the position. Announcing the establishment of the position was one thing. Making it functional was quite another. The consensus both within and outside the department was that the proposal should be allowed to go through because it would eventually die a natural death like most political gimmicks. And that is precisely what happened. The Department of Health's opposition had achieved one important goal. It had stalled the proposal long enough for people to have doubts about it and up to the time when the governor had to announce who he was supporting in the mayoral race. Eventually the governor did what we hoped he would, support someone other than Beame. That insured the end of the health czar proposal.

THE FINAL PROPOSAL

On March 28, 1977, Governor Carey and Mayor Beame made public a memorandum of understanding concerning the Director and Coordinator of Health for New York City. It read as follows:

Section 1. The director will be jointly appointed by the governor and the mayor. This shall be a temporary position. This position is required because of the obvious need to address urgent problems in the health care delivery system that are now under state, city and federal jurisdiction.

To accomplish the goals and responsibilities listed below, the director shall serve as the principal health advisor to the mayor and shall have vested in him all the necessary responsibilities by the state to fulfill his task. He shall report directly to the assistant to the governor for health afffairs and the first deputy mayor. The New York City Commissioner of Health shall report to the director with respect to hospitals, ambulatory care and all health care delivery matters.

The governor and the mayor will ask the Board of Directors of the Health Systems Agency of New York City to make the director chairman of its executive committee in lieu of the Commissioner of Health.

Section 2. In the city of New York, the director shall:

a. Plan, coordinate and direct New York City health operations as they relate to the goals and responsibilities listed below.

b. Develop a responsive health care structure and resource capability to deal effectively with the rapidly changing demands for health care services in New York City.

c. Plan innovative cost effective improvements to reduce operating expenses and minimize the need for additional capital or human resources in the delivery of health care.

d. Review and approve the financial plan (as well as the location and type of services and facilities) of the NYC Health and Hospitals Corporation before these are submitted by the city to the Emergency Financial Control Board.

e. Serve as Health Services Administrator/Chairman of Board of Directors of the New York City Health and Hospitals Corporation for the purposes of the goals and responsibilities listed below.

f. Act as Chairman of the Inter-Agency Health Council which shall consist of the commissioners of Health, Mental Health, Addiction Services, and Social Services, the President of the Health and Hospitals

Corporation, and the Director of Management and Budget. The Executive Director of the Health Systems Agency will be invited to participate on the Inter-Agency Health Council.

g. Serve as permanent alternate for the Commissioner of Health on the board and executive committee of the Health Systems Agency of New York City until the HSA by-laws are changed.

Section 3. For the State of New York, the director shall:

a. Serve as deputy commissioner of health for New York City Affairs. The New York State Commissioner of Health shall delegate to the Director the power to decertify beds and all necessary powers relating to the health care delivery system as they relate to New York City.

b. Serve as deputy director of the State Health Planning Commission and be delegated all of the responsibilities and functions of that Commission in New York City.

Section 4. Goals and Responsibilities
Specifically the director will:

a. Develop, identify, and institute policies to:
    i.   Consolidate the institutional system of health care delivery by eliminating unneeded facilities and unused capacity. This shall apply to the municipal, voluntary and proprietary hospital systems as well as the long-term care facilities.
    ii. Improve the efficiency of the health care delivery system by eliminating duplicative services, and by encouraging the development of ambulatory services and other alternate and more cost-effective forms of care.
    iii. Establish a regional system of health care so that access to the reduced system is guaranteed to those in need of medical care.

b. Serve as the City's and State's liaison with the Federal government on policy matters relating to the reimbursement of health care services in the City of New York.

    c.   Review and comment on all systems used for regulating and financing the health care system in New York City to ensure that these are consistent with a consolidated system able to provide necessary health care.

    d.   Reshape existing regulatory programs to clearly delineate responsibility, reduce administrative costs, and ensure an effective review of providers to protect the interests of the State/City and the recipients of care.

Section 5. Staffing And Offices

The Director and his staff shall receive joint support from the City and State. It is estimated that a staff of 10-15 professional level people will be required, some of which can be transferred from existing lines on the City and State level. The Director shall have office space similar to that assigned to Deputy Mayors.

THE AFTERMATH

The joint mayoral and gubernatorial announcement received a great deal of attention in the press.[37-41] Then for the next two weeks nothing more was heard. Behind the scenes, Cahill had embarked on what would prove to be an unsuccessful attempt to get a highly qualified person to take the position. Finally, on April 12, 1977, the board of the Health Systems Agency passed a resolution condemning the whole concept of a health czar.[42] The deputy executive director of the agency related that there was enough power in already existing state and city agencies to carry out what was needed and that the health czar merely represented another layer of bureaucracy.[43] The *Amsterdam News* had earlier condemned the health czar concept.[44] The Health Systems Agency may have balked at the health commissioner as chairman of its executive committee. But a health czar partially appointed by the governor was a far more threatening possibility.

Failure to expeditiously find someone for the position made it difficult to recruit a replacement for the outgoing HHC president, due to leave on April 30.[45] Obviously, no one wanted to accept the HHC presidency without knowing who would be the health czar and how this person would act in his or her numerous capacities. In

order to provide the HHC with some kind of leadership after Holloman's departure, the board acted on a proposal made by the mayor's
office to establish a special eight-person Interim Operating Committee with Donald Kummerfeld, then director of the mayor's Office of
Management and Budget as chairman.[46-49] In addition, the mayor,
Zuccotti, and Kummerfeld later proposed that the board name
Joseph Lynaugh, then the executive director of the Health Systems
Agency and Le Roy Carmichael, executive director of Queens Hospital Center as executive vice-president.[50] Thus, the mayor tightened
his grip on the corporation. Although certain board members
engaged in vocal protests for the benefit of diverse constituencies, a
majority went along with these proposals. For it had become clear to
them that the board had run out of options in extricating the HHC
from its financial troubles.

Meanwhile, as Lynaugh and Carmichael were being confirmed
in their new positions, the governor announced the creation of the
cabinet-level Office of Health Systems Management.[51] This office
assumed the state health department's role setting, regulatory, and
Medicaid auditing functions.

The search for a health czar continued, and on May 12, 1977,
the *New York Daily News* reported that Dr. Cahill was down to four
candidates, but that the job was in peril.[52] The four were thought to
be too closely linked to certain political interests to enable them to
proceed with hospital closures. Then, in June Governor Carey threw
his support behind Mario Cuomo, the state's Secretary of State in the
latter's bid for the Democratic Party's nomination for mayor. One of
the principal reasons for the mayor's support of the proposal was no
longer operative, and he suddenly cooled to the whole idea.[53] John
Zuccotti left office on June 30, 1977 to enter private life and was
replaced as first deputy mayor by Donald Kummerfeld.[54] Kummerfeld pubicly stated that he wanted to take a long, hard look at the
health czar proposal before negotiating with Dr. Cahill. Both Cahill
and Zuccotti denied that the political fallout between Carey and
Beame had resulted in the latter's backing away from the proposal.[55]
However, it was clear to many close to the issue that this indeed was
what had happened. As far as Mayor Beame was concerned, the
health czar proposal was a dead issue.

On June 9, 1977, the HHC board voted to name Joseph
Lynaugh as acting president, thus giving the mayor considerable
control over the corporation.

Finally, in September Dr. Cahill renewed his efforts with Mayor Beame on a joint state-city health czar. Beame was uninterested in the proposal. By this time he had lost the Democratic nomination, the winner being Congressman Edward I. Koch, who beat the governor's candidate, Mario Cuomo, in a runoff. Koch, certain to win the November election, did not rush to endorse the proposal either, saying that he needed more time to study it.[56]

In September 1977, Governor Carey announced his appointment of a health czar. Because of the city's refusal to participate, the candidate was, as one official put it, only half a czar.[57] Carey's choice, Morton Hyman, was a millionaire shipping executive who had served for a number of years as a member of the State Public Health Council, the counterpart of the city's Board of Health.[58] The governor presented Hyman as a Medicaid expert because of his having chaired a council subcommittee dealing with Medicaid matters. But whether Hyman possessed the needed administrative skills and knowledge to operationally implement his sweeping mandate was an open question for most public health authorities. This, however, was of little concern to city officials because the appointment had no practical significance for them. And within several months, the entire health czar issue faded from the scene.

AN ASSESSMENT

As a case study, New York State's health czar proposal of 1977 illustrates a number of important points with regard to health services administration. Although designed by a professional, its intent was purely political, serving the interests of a governor who wanted a shelter from unpopular decisions. While elected political leaders enjoy their authorities and powers, they invariably avoid using them to make decisions which, while in the best interests of all, carry significant adverse political consequences. Hospital closure and service reductions were certainly unpopular prospects for blocks of voters, particularly hospital workers and communities served by hospitals. Yet they were viewed as necessary to the maintenance of the city's fiscal health. No governor or mayor likes to be associated with such unpopular decisions, even though they have the authority to make them through their appointed officials. Thus, in order to make the health czar proposal seem reasonable, the governor and his special assistant for health affairs had to construct a convincing case for the governor's lack of such authority and for its genesis through a process of job consolidation. As convincing as all this may have sounded to the general public, the experts were not fooled by it for one moment.

The proposal was made possible in part by the erosion of the healthy checks and balances that had once existed between state and local government. The driving engines of this erosion were the fiscal crisis, which stripped the city of its remaining autonomy, and a conscious state policy of progressive centralization. Thus, the ground was fertile for the commission of political excesses. While incrementalism characterizes decision-making processes in structures with healthy checks and balances, quantum leaps frequently reflect an excess of centralized power. The health czar proposal was a reflection of such centralized power. The proposal was presented to the city as a non-negotiable public policy, a state posture that would not have been possible a few years before when the city's autonomy was still intact. Despite repeated attempts, reasoned opinion failed to sway the proposal's architects.

Mayor Beame, and John Zuccotti, the first deputy mayor, were weakened in their resolve to resist because of the former's need of gubernatorial support in the upcoming mayoral election. Of no small interest is the fact that the mayor dropped all interest in the matter as soon as the governor threw his political support to a rival candidate. Beame obviously knew that he had a difficult uphill fight ahead to win reelection particularly since so many unjustly associated him in a cause and effect manner with the fiscal crisis. His willingness to endorse the health czar proposal in exchange for potential gubernatorial support demonstrated the vulnerability of his political position. For this was a mayor who had otherwise given an enormous degree of support to an independent city health department. Put succinctly, his willingness to endorse a proposal as ill conceived as the health czar was, frankly, out of character for him.

As explained above, the office of the health czar was poorly conceived and flew in the face of basic administrative wisdom. In reality, the person in the position would have had a line relationship to the city's first deputy mayor, also a line position to the state's health commissioner, since he would have been a deputy health commissioner for New York City affairs, and to the governor's special health advisor, who was in a staff position. It is difficult to imagine that the position could work under three separate superordinates. Additionally, as chairman of the executive committee of the city's Health Systems Agency and simultaneously deputy director of the state's Health Planning Commission, the health czar would have been in an untenable situation, since the latter had ratification powers over the decisions of the former. Similarly, other positions, such as the chairmanship of the HHC board, would have placed the incumbent into direct conflict with his other roles.

Some have cogently argued that the consolidation of positions represented by the health czar was an attempt to remove the system of checks and balances between the positions, it being perceived that they stood in the way of decisive action. The first postulate rings true, but the latter does not, since the statutory authorities for health care facilities closure rested with the state health commissioner and the certificate of need process, which allows facilities to open and operate with the governor's special health advisor. When all is said and done, the needed authorities were there, but with a governor who feared the political consequences of their use. So, in the final analysis, one comes back to the fact that the proposal was politically motivated.

The inclusion of the New York City Department of Health in the proposal seemed almost gratuitous because the department had absolutely no hospital functions. By insisting that the city health commissioner report to the health czar, Cahill was, in effect, reducing the commissionership to a position below that of a deputy commissioner in the state health department. For the health czar was to be simultaneously a deputy health commissioner of the state health department and, in that capacity, the superordinate of the city health commissioner. The leadership of the city health department could have meekly accepted the proposal and subsequently witnessed the denigration and dismantling of the department, or they could have resisted. They chose to resist. This option by definition brought them into immediate conflict with the governor's special health advisor who was by then the most powerful health official in the state, having already brought the state health commissioner to heel. It subsequently created a confrontation with city officials as well, who, desirous of currying the governor's support for the mayor's reelection bid, were willing to go along with the proposal.

The decision to resist was made quickly and decisively, and with full knowledge of the consequences. The principal consequence was job loss. This option was preferable to the department's leadership over job retention, because the latter would have meant presiding over the department's decline. The secondary consequences were weeks of badgering and cajoling by state and city officials and criticism by those segments of the press that rushed to support the proposal either out of personal or political loyalty to the govenor or out of a sincere belief in its worth. For public health physicians who were eminently reemployable elsewhere in better paying positions and under better working conditions, resistance was not a difficult option. This resistance centered around myself because I was the health commissioner. But it was shared by my top staff and eventually supported by the Board of Health.

What eventually slowed the state-city process down was my own threat of resignation. Mayor Beame may have been willing to accept a health czar, albeit reluctantly, but not at the price of losing his health commissioner. Slowing the process down gave time for a larger event to play itself out, namely, the governor's choosing of a mayoral candidate. He inadvertently did the cause of public health a service by supporting one of the mayor's rivals because this led to mayoral abandonment of the entire proposal.

Although the Department of Health emerged victorious from this protracted struggle, it did not do so undamaged. Having been the object of consideration for structural and governance changes that would have removed its independence, eroded its functions, and denigrated its general position, the department was correctly perceived as potentially vulnerable to renewed attack. This blocked the inflow of younger professionals unsure of the department's future, and had a demoralizing effect on existing staff. The health commissioner's effectiveness with the HHC and the Health Systems Agency was greatly damaged as the newspapers discussed his removal from posts under a health czar. And his relationships with numerous extra-departmental groups and organizations were damaged because, in the minds of many, the health department had an uncertain future under a health czar.

In retrospect, the health czar proposal got as far as it did because of a confluence of political and fiscal circumstances, the absence of the usual checks and balances between the state and a locality, and the concentration of power with regard to health affairs in the hands of a staff person responsible to no one but the governor. The proposal was ultimately abadoned, and its chief architect eventually resigned.[59,60]

Chapter 13

DEALING WITH THE PRESS
AND MEDIA

While traditional modalities of public health education have an important place, they pale next to the impact that can be achieved through the press and media when a newsworthy problem arises. For experienced public health officials know not only how to discuss the problem, but also how to take advantage of its presence. The sudden appearance of even one diagnosed case of diphtheria in New York City is cause for headlines because the disease is of such low incidence. A Commissioner of Health should not only discuss the problem but should also raise the issue of childhood immunization and its importance in preventing disease.

Dealing with the press and media in a city with a hundred A.M. and F.M. radio stations, seven television stations, and numerous newspapers requires not only sound technical knowledge but an ability to use it on camera and over the radio at a moment's notice. It also requires an ability to state highly complex and technical problems in words understandable to the average layman.

Health officials must acquaint themselves with how the media operate and, in return for cooperating, will receive high levels of reward for the cause of public health. They must come to realize that what is crucial to the media and press is not only what is said and how it is said, but when it is said as well. A health official who puts off calls from radio stations and refuses television crew access to his office achieves one sure objective. He leaves it to others to interpret the situation and in so doing runs the risk of their doing so inaccurately. What is said by a health commissioner at 3 P.M. may have no impact if it should have been said at 10:00 A.M. The ability to respond in an immediate manner requires knowledge, ability, and decisiveness. Health officials must come to realize that aside from the inherent competitiveness in the communications business, reporters face practical problems—type for the morning papers is set by late afternoon and film footage for evening television news broadcasts cut by 4 P.M.

There are a number of public health officials who either consciously or subconsciously assign a low priority to telling the press and media what is happening. In their view, they have the problem in hand and are satisfied it is on the way to resolution. This may be the reality, but if the press and media are not told about it it will not be the reality perceived by the public. Events affecting the public health are not like the procedures and results of laboratory experiments that can be kept secret at will. The public has a right to know, and public health officials who interpret this as a privilege eventually bring themselves to grief.

DIRECTING PUBLIC RELATIONS

Because of the size of the New York City Department of Health, the scope of its functions, and the frequency of press and media interest in its activities, a full-time public relations director has been in a staff position under the Commissioner of Health for many years. The individuals who have occupied this position have generally been of superior quality and have usually had an excellent working knowledge of the New York City press corps and the media. Many brought long-standing personal relationships with people in the press and media to the position as well.

The first step in public relations is the establishment of departmental structure and policies. And the second is the execution of press relations policies. The two commonest models used by health departments are for the chief executive to direct public relations or for a full-time director working under a chief executive to do so. It is the latter model that has been used in the New York City health department.

Such a director drafts regular press releases, maintains ongoing contact with the press and media, arranges guest appearances for the commissioner or other departmental officials on radio and television, and operationally directs all of the department's contacts with the press and media. There is great value in all such contacts being cleared through a public relations director and, conversely, great jeopardy in not doing so.

THE CHOICE OF SPOKESMEN

A common mistake made by public health agencies is to allow more than one person on the staff to comment to the press on a given problem. Assuming there is no controversy within the agency on the handling of a problem, and in my experience this rarely arose in the New York City Health Department, there should be only one spokesman. If there is more than one spokesman, the following scenario develops. Spokesman One says, "the situation should be under control in two to three days." Spokesman Two says, "the problem will be largely solved in about four days or so." And Spokesman Three says, "the problem will be over in a week." Professionals have enough knowledge and insight to realize there are no contradictions in these statements. Journalists may not, and it is almost a certainty that the public will be confused. Also, the use of different technical nuances is vulnerable to the creation of controversy and confusion where none need exist.

"Who knows what's going on?" the average layman will ask. But this is not the more serious, long-lasting effect of such poor handling of public relations. The agency will be perceived as confused, and the public made to wonder who is really in charge.

All of this can be averted by having one spokesman who answer all of the questions from the press and media. This spokesman can be either the staff person in charge of the general area into which the problem falls or the head of the agency. Public relations directors play a crucial role in assisting either of these two individuals in a variety of ways. But they should not be cast in the role of spokesman. The credibility of what is said about health problems is enhanced by the professional qualifications and authoritativeness of the spokesman.

Frequently, when directors of public relations speak for an agency, they are being used by agency heads as a protective screen from embarrassing issues. The frequent use of this device for this purpose is widely known not only to journalists, but also to large segments of the listening, viewing, and reading public. This alone is sufficient reason for not using it. And indeed, most New York City health commissioners have avoided it.

Some health commissioners have chosen to be the almost exclusive spokesmen for most issues. This has the advantage of resulting in a consistent response to all queries on a given issue. A commissioner responding to a dozen successive telephone calls from radio stations and newspaper journalists is less likely to produce nuances of difference that could be construed as confusing than are several spokesmen speaking separately but simultaneously.

The disadvantage of this approach is that program directors and subordinates whose technical expertise may have resulted in program successes do not get into the limelight. And this can lead to the development of resentments against commissioners who consistently exclude them from press and media exposure. Commissioners, on the other hand, must maintain an image of leadership consistency not only in departmental policies, but also in their presentation to the public. Many have viewed the resentment of subordinates over this issue as a small price to pay given their responsiveness to subordinates in other areas that enhance job satisfaction.

In part, the problem can be dealt with by the commissioner maintaining his role as chief spokesman but permitting appropriate subordinates to enhance and elaborate upon a story with specific details. And, indeed, this was the approach used during Dr. Lowell Bellin's commissionership and my own. Press releases were worded so that the commissioner made the announcement of a new finding, the appearance of a new problem, or the results of a program, followed by quotes from program directors in which details were spelled out. This resulted in press and media stories in which attribution was given to both the commissioner and specific subordinates. This permitted the commissioner to maintain his leadership position in the public eye while at the same time giving recognition and satisfaction to his subordinates.

Commissioners who shun the press and the media and who consistently allow subordinates and directors of public relations to be spokesmen project a poor leadership image. Not infrequently, this public image has been an accurate reflection of reality.

PRESS CONFERENCES AND MEETINGS WITH THE PRESS AND MEDIA

Although press conferences are still an important forum for announcing news of different kinds, they are not for the New York City Department of Health. The decline of the press conference modality for the health department can be traced to technological advances and news producer attitudes. As far as news producers and managers are concerned, health commissioners rarely have announcements to make that are so important as to require their sending reporters to cover them at a specified time. Limited reporter staff has to be spread thin to cover the major, breaking stories. However, media and press managers are always interested in health department news and invariably cover it. Generally they prefer that their reporters individualize interviews. This is important to them because of its impact on program ratings. Similarly, it is important to reporters who can demonstrate reportorial abilities, insights, and investigative skills through the individualized interview.

Because of technological advances, radio interviews can be obtained over the telephone and television stations can send crews out at their convenience to record an interview. Likewise, print journalists can conduct their interviews over the phone at their convenience. Thus, the usual pattern in New York City is for the media and press to descend on the health department when a story is released or news is breaking at unpredictable intervals via phone and in person. Because of this, it is crucial to have a good director of public relations who can properly schedule the visits and organize the telephone interviews.

Feature stories and discussions of departmental policies and programs are often handled on talk shows and at scheduled interviews, either at the health department or at studios or newspaper headquarters. Often, health department officials are invited for interviews not about specific New York City problems but about national ones because the media and press wish to draw upon the expertise and authoritativeness of given public health experts. Such interviews may be scheduled in advance. But in a crisis situation, the media and press approach the health department in much the same way they do when a story is breaking in the city.

SERVING AS A RESOURCE

Quite frequently, press and media journalists contact health department officials in order to obtain different types of technical information. Although these requests come from a variety of journalists, they are most frequently made by science and health reporters in the process of putting together a special story. They request not only specific technical information, but also leads about where to contact specialists and where to unearth published materials. In responding to these requests, departmental staff serve as an information resource and enable the press and media to achieve their goals. Because the department and its staff are often not involved in the final program, nor given public acknowledgement, the argument has been raised that the service should not be provided.

This position is shortsighted, in my view, because providing this kind of help expands and solidifies relationships between the department and the press and media. In turn, they have consistently responded to departmental requests for disseminating important public health messages and information about public health programs.

THE DETERMINANTS OF PRESS AND MEDIA COVERAGE

The Department of Health does not obtain press and media coverage by simply putting out press releases. And those who view health commissioners or other departmental officials who frequently make the news as publicity seekers betray their woeful ignorance of how the press and media operate. For a story to get into print, it must be newsworthy. And to be newsworthy, a story must be either topical, important, controversial or sensational. If it does not possess one of these characteristics, it is unlikely to become a major news item.

Departmental news releases about the risk of heat stroke and heat exhaustion, for example, invariably make local headlines during July heat waves. The same releases, if put out on a cool spring day, would be ignored. An announcement of a rise in the number of heroin addicts in the city is newsworthy no matter the magnitude of the rise. But a news release describing a slight fall in such numbers would be ignored. The issues surrounding the 1976 swine influenza immunization program were treated with banner headlines because they were controversial. News release information about routine departmental childhood immunization programs rarely gets into print. Similarly, one case of diphtheria in the city is sensational and makes headlines, whereas ten thousand cases of gonorrhea are viewed as routine and are ignored by the press and media.

Exposure of the department and its officials in the press and media does not depend solely on what takes place in New York City. Commissioners and their staff with proven knowledge, recognized expertise, and stage presence are often called upon to comment on national issues and problems. For example, officials in the department were widely quoted in the city's papers when the Chinese conducted an atmospheric nuclear test in 1977. There was great concern in the United States about atomic fallout and its effects on the public health. Similar coverage has been given to the department subsequent to newsworthy announcements made by federal health agencies and national medical groups. But all such coverage is dependent on the presence of knowledgeable and articulate experts in the department.

Some public health officials are given more media coverage than others, not just because they are spokesmen for newsworthy issues. The media tend to call upon experts who have both proven stage presence and an ability to explain complex technical matters in laymen's terms. So often, those who possess expert knowledge cannot communicate it in simple, direct language. Their statements are full of jargon and technical terms, understandable only to other experts. Media journalists tend to shun the future interviewing of such people. This deficiency on the part of public health experts, physicians especially, results from years of communication in exclusively technical language. Additionally, some public health officials have a pejorative attitude toward the press and media and view their inquiries as probes to be repulsed by the techniques of evasion and no comment. Others are uncomfortable on stage and go to any lengths to avoid looking into a television camera, even if the stage be their own office. I recall an eminent public health physician in a nearby health department who fled his office whenever he heard that a television film crew was on its way.

Surprisingly, there are some public health officials who pride themselves on avoiding contacts with the press and media. These officials also demonstrate a certain consistency in never taking a public stand on any thing, especially controversial issues. In so doing they drift into a comfortable backwater, which is viable until some spirited public official begins to wonder about what the local health department is doing. In adopting this course of action they make themselves and their departments vulnerable to a variety of adverse consequences, including budgetary ones. For, it is not only important that a health department do its job well, but equally important that the public know it. In the final analysis, reality is the reality that is perceived by most and not necessarily the reality that is. It is a public health official's task to see to it that the latter is perceived.

It is often easier for a public health official to achieve anonymity and the luxury of privacy while in public office than for a flamboyant publicity seeker to get constant exposure. The press and media avoid the lacklusters and tend to leave unwilling health officials alone. Insulation is further insured by failure to put out frequent press releases, by being unavailable for comment or by deferring comment until after the peak of interest has passed.

Publicity-seeking public health officials do occasionally succeed in obtaining coverage because they are adept at presenting issues and problems as surrogates of themselves. Standing in favor of success for these individuals is their frequent espousal of controversial positions on important issues. However, the press and media are not always the easy instruments of such people and often exercise a healthy scrutiny of their claims and statements. Although they may gain notoriety, in the process such individuals usually erode their credibility. This results in their publicity seeking not having much staying power.

MAYORAL CLEARANCE

In principal, the Commissioner of Health, as a mayoral appointee, is a member of the executive branch and must support the administration's overall policies or leave office. It has been rare for mayors to make quantum changes in policies, the notable example being during the Beame administration when impending municipal bankruptcy forced such changes. In general, mayors have press secretaries who quickly establish a relationship with departmental public relations directors. During the Beame administration, the Director of Public Information of the health department did not report directly to the mayor's press secretary, but to the health commissioner. They did, however, have an excellent working relationship and frequently communicated on diverse matters.

During the Beame administration, press releases put out by the health department did not have to receive prior approval by the mayor's press secretary, because most releases dealt with technical, medical, and public health subjects. However, the mayor's press secretary was routinely consulted whenever the department publicly dealt with important policy matters and political issues. Such consultation often resulted in valuable assistance.

Of note is the fact that the reporters who covered municipal government events at city hall from Room Nine, the press room, rarely dealt with the health department. Science, health, and medical reporters working from their home offices were the journalists who usually covered the department. Consequently, health department officials often interacted with journalists the mayor's press secretary hardly knew.

Highly controversial political matters were often handled directly by the mayor's press secretary working in concert with the department's public information director. This allowed for a unified and consistent administration stand, a characteristic often lacking even in the federal government, where the White House must often clarify statements made by various departmental secretaries. The press and media are quick to read controversy and opinion difference into statements made independently by members of the same administration because this makes news. To avoid this, and the nightmare of making endless clarifying statements, a unified stand was generally made at the outset. Obviously, this process did not pertain to situations in which the mayor and a commissioner were at odds over policy. But public confrontation over policy was rare.

Mayoral aides were not above giving leaks or planting stories in order to bring a recalcitrant commissioner around to their way of thinking. This occurred during the health czar crisis of 1977 (see Chapter 12). Similarly, mayoral aides and press secretaries often issue important press releases covering controversial matters and reflecting policy decisions opposed by commissioners on holidays and Sundays. This has a two-fold effect. Most press and media journalists are off and not around to ask potentially embarrassing questions. By the time they return, the item is no longer newsworthy. Commissioners are caught off guard and are unable to mount effective opposition. Wise commissioners do not generally take vacations or go away for long weekends when the mayor or mayoral aides are contemplating policy decisions adverse to their departments. For if they do, they will find the matter resolved against them when they return.

Clearly, the relationship between health commissioners nad mayors has not been a consistently cooperative one. There have been periods of conflict, preferably kept out of the public view, and sometimes serious confrontations. A free hand was given by Mayor Beame to his health commissioners in dealing with the press and media on professional and technical matters. But firmer mayoral control was understandably exercised when it came to major public policy issues.

CREDIBILITY OF THE PRESS AND MEDIA

At the dawn of the 1980s, it was clear that both the press and media had lost credibility with vast segments of the public.[1] As *U.S. News and World Report* succinctly stated, print journalism was under attack, with widespread charges of fabricated stories, inaccurate reporting, and lax editing.[2] The competition with television felt by print journalists has been a major factor in escalating abuses that have been present for many years. For its part, television has not been above criticism for fabrications, distortions, over dramatizations, and selective editing.

Another important factor that has led to an increase in these abuses is the so called "new journalism" that emerged during the social upheaval of the late 1960s. The essence of this form of journalism is the use of composite characters, the reporting of dialogue and events not personally witnessed, and the recounting of the innermost thoughts of subjects.[3] When used together, these techniques can lead to gross distortions and, in the hands of ambitious, unscrupulous, or careless individuals, to dishonest reporting.[4]

Government officials, the individuals most often exposed to press and media scrutiny and the frequent victims of dishonest journalism, have long known of these abuses. However, since the late 1970s the general public has had its confidence in television and print news eroded as it has grown steadily aware of these abuses. In 1981, two well-publicized instances of dishonest reporting only served to confirm the general public's silent majority opinion, "You can't believe what you read in the papers." The first concerned a Pulitzer Prize winning story about an eight-year-old heroin addict. This story, which ran in the *Washington Post*, was pure fabrication and led to the resignation of the reporter and the return of the prize. Interestingly, the returned prize was then given to a reporter for the *Village Voice* whose stories included one about the accused killer of former Representative Allard Lowenstein of New York. A journalist from another New York paper charged that the story gave the misleading impression that a personal interview had taken place. The charge was sustained by the National News Council.[5]

In 1981, a *New York Daily News* journalist resigned after he could not substantiate portions of an article he had written about Northern Ireland. He admitted that he had used a fictitious name for the story's central figure.[6] In Oregon, an associate editor of the *Portland Oregonian* admitted he fabricated quotes that he attributed to then Governor Dixy Lee Ray of Washington.[7] The editor was suspended for sixty days.

On October 5, 1981, the *Washington Post* gossip column, "The Ear," printed a story that accused the Carter White House of bugging the Blair House conversations of President-elect and Mrs. Reagan. Former President Carter and Mrs. Carter threatened to sue the newspaper for libel.[8] They demanded a retraction and an apology the day the item appeared.[9] Nine days later, on October 14, 1981, the paper ran an editorial in which it admitted that the eavesdropping report was "utterly impossible to believe."[10] However, the editors did not admit that they had erred in printing the story. During the nine-day period between the original story and the editorial, matters were worsened by statements made by staff members of the Post. On October 8, Dianna McClellan, the journalist who wrote the gossip column, said the Carters knew perfectly well that the story was true.[11] And Benjamin C. Bradlee, executive editor of the paper, tried to trivialize the matter by saying of the former President's demand for an apology, "How do you make an apology—run up and down Pennsylvania Avenue shouting, I'm sorry?"[12]

What troubled Mr. Carter and many others concerned with the integrity of the press was the Post's claim in its October 14 editorial to have the right to publish rumors that are damaging to innocent people even if the paper's editors believe them to be untrue.[13] The editorial said: "Perhaps it is foolish to expect people to read newspapers with rabbinical or juridical care, to sift out the fair from the unfair or the justified from the unjustified inferences that can be drawn from a collection of words."[14]

Finally, on October 23, 1981, two and a half weeks after the story appeared, Post publisher Donald E. Graham sent Mr. and Mrs. Carter a letter of apology, retracting the false allegation and stating that the *Washington Post* does not claim the right to print rumors without verification of their accuracy.[15]

Mr. Carter, in his statement about Graham's letter of apology and retraction, made an extremely cogent point. He said: ''...because of my previous position, I had access to the public news media and could draw attention to my problem. Many victims of similarly false allegations do not enjoy this opportunity, but suffer just as severely.''[16] Although newspapers regularly print letters from readers, it is worth noting that most of these letters either challenge editorials or state views. Newspapers rarely print letters that challenge the accuracy of their news stories. To do so exposes them to an erosion of public confidence. And this can ultimately lead to falling sales and fiscal insolvency. What Mr. Carter was saying was that many people who are severely wronged by inaccurate newspaper stories usually cannot undo the damage. The offending paper will not run a correcting letter of protest, and other papers, protective of their brethren, are unlikely to do so either. It is of interest, for example, that *The New York Times*, in reporting the *Washington Post's* final retraction, did so on pages 26 and 27 of a large and bulky Sunday edition. Some would cogently argue that a story of this importance should have appeared somewhere between pages 1 and 3. Instead, it was buried away in the depths of the paper.

These well-publicized instances have not only fueled public skepticism about journalistic honesty, but have also tarnished the image of the Pulitzer Prize. Some critics of the press and media have gone so far as to say that most events are routinely underreported, overreported, or misreported.[17] On the positive side, these events, and increasing doubts about press and media credibility, have led to an acceleration of standard setting and control processes by editors of papers that had already begun to institute remedial measures, as well as the initiation of such measures by a number of other editors. Many editors are now exercising tighter control over reporters and are issuing guidelines on acceptable practices.[18] The National News Council, a watchdog organization, was established in the 1970s to deal with complaints about journalism and to examine issues concerning press standards. It is funded in part by press organizations.[19]

As good as all these measures are, they are unable to completely remedy abuses that can catapult a dishonest journalist to a page one byline and advance his career. It is not unreasonable to assume that these abuses will continue to exist, to some degree, for a long time to come. Therefore, public health officials and others must prepare to not only complain about them, but more important, to raise their defenses against them.

Some of the techniques currently used by journalists whose stories would fail to pass acceptable press standards include fabrications, embellishments, intentional distortions, framing questions, editorializing on the news pages, characterizing people and feelings on scanty evidence, using quotes out of context, or else selectively sustaining preconceived or contrived story lines. Such reporters can also hide behind the screen of anonymous sources or so called "informed sources' in writing a story.

Public health officials can protect themselves against some of these techniques by using both common sense and specific countermeasures. As a general rule, it is always prudent for interviews to be given in the presence of one or two senior colleagues. The presence of such witnesses has a two-fold effect. It can curtail journalistic abuse in some instances, and constitutes an invaluable resource in redressing abuse once it has occurred. Journalists with a proven history of inaccurate or distorted reporting are simply best avoided, as are those who are strongly committed to a particular point of view opposed to of the interviewee. In either instance, it is virtually assumed that the interviewee and his policy decisions or positions will emerge in a bad light.

Questions should be answered carefully and thoughtfully and not with off-handed remarks. Breezy comments should never be made. Many an interviewee has been pained to find such comments in print in the next day's paper. It is a healthy defensive strategy for public health officials to learn how to evade leading and framed questions. Skilled journalists know how to draw out the answers they are seeking, and those being interviewed must become as skilled in not falling into such traps.

The use by television news programs of videotape poses special hazards in the hands of dishonest journalists or editors.' Tapes can be cut to convey totally different meanings than those intended by the person interviewed. This can easily be accomplished, for example, by cutting and then splicing the response to one question after another. For this reason, a number of public figures will give only live interviews.

Television journalists may lure an unsuspecting individual into circumstances they perceive as providing either drama or confrontation. There was one local television news journalist in New York City, for example, who would ask officials to come out onto the sidewalk for interviews, claiming malfunctioning lighting equipment. Once there he would surface a preselected "average citizen" who allegedly was just passing by and invite him to confront the official on a currently controversial issue. This journalist also engaged in the "ambush interview,' in which he would arrive unannounced and start questioning a startled official while the cameras were rolling. It is easy to understand the genesis of such abuses in light of the fact that many television news journalists and editors see entertainment as an important part of their mission. This has been fueled by the felt need to score well in ratings and best rivals. And there is no denying that the entertainment components of news broadcasts attract viewers. Some have cogently argued that entertainment has not role in news reporting.

Newspapers and television news programs are keenly aware of the public's loss of confidence in them. In 1980, an ABC-Hams Survey disclosed that only 29 percent of the public had a great deal of confidence in television news. For print news the figure was 19 percent.[20] Coupled with this low level of credibility is a high level of public resentment and anger over the perceived arrogance and power of the press and media. Journalistic leaders have interpreted these ominous realities correctly and have made moves to regain public confidence. The effectiveness of their reform measures has still to be evaluated, and only time will determine whether they have staying power. Meanwhile, all public health officials must continue to deal with a press and media corps whose quality is uneven and whose honesty and integrity are sometimes in doubt.

REFERENCE NOTES

CHAPTER 1

1. W.S. Sayre and H. Kaufman, *Governing New York City: Politics In the Metropolis* (New York: Russell Sage Foundation, 1960), p. 26.
2. N. Glazer and D.P. Moynihan, *Beyond the Melting Pot* (Cambridge, Ma: MIT Press and Harvard University Press), 1963.
3. K. Auletta, *The Streets Were Paved With Gold* (New York: Random House, 1979), pp. 3-27.
4. P.J. Imperato, "Current Problems of Some New York City Health Agencies," *Bulletin of the New York Academy of Medicine* (1979), 55(5), pp. 463-476.
5. U.S. Bureau of the Census. *Characteristics of the Population*, Volume 1, Part 34, *New York*, Section 1, Washington, D.C. U.S.G.P.O., 1971.
6. Ibid., Tables 9, 125, and 129.
7. Census Indicates A Sharp Decline In Whites In City, *New York Times* (April 6, 1981), pp. 1, B6.
8. Auletta, *The Streets Were Paved With Gold*, pp. 11-12.
9. C.L. Morris, *The Cost of Good Intentions: New York City and The Liberal Experiment, 1960-1975* (New York, Norton), 1980, p. 140.
10. Auletta, *The Streets Were Paved With Gold*, pp. 11-12.
11. Morris, *The Cost of Good Intentions*, p. 140.
12. Ibid., p. 141.
13. Ibid.
14. Ibid.
15. Auletta, *The Streets Were Paved With Gold*, pp. 19-20.
16. Ibid., p. 20.
17. F.S. Kristoff, "Housing: Facets of New York City's Problems," in *Agenda For A City: Confronting New York*, L.C. Fitch and A.H. Kauk, eds. (New York: Institute of Public Administration, 1970), pp. 197-325.

18. Auletta, *The Streets Were Paved With Gold*, p. 15.
19. Kristoff, "Housing: Facets of New York City's Problems."
20. Auletta, *The Streets Were Paved With Gold*, p. 143.
21. Ibid.
22. *Public Assistance Programs in New York City*, (New York: The Temporary Commission on City Finances), 1977.
23. E.J. Kennedy, Speech To The Twenty-Third Annual NAACP Dinner, Detroit, May, 1978.
24. Auletta, *The Streets Were Paved With Gold*, p. 194.
25. P.J. Imperato, "The Effect of New York City's Fiscal Crisis on the Department of Health," *Bulletin of the New York Academy of Medicine*, 54(3), pp. 276-289, 1978.
26. Auletta, *The Streets Were Paved With Gold*, pp. 3-27.
27. N. Hentoff, *A Political Life: The Education of John V. Lindsay* (New York: Knopf, 1969).
28. City In Crisis, series in the *New York Herald Tribune*, New York, January 24, 1965 through February 18, 1965.
29. J.R. Dumpson, "Aiding the City's Poor," *Governing The City: Challenges and Options for New York*, edited by R.H. Connery and D. Caraley, eds., New York: Praeger, 1969), pp. 148-161.
30. Morris, *The Cost of Good Intentions*, pp. 20-21.
31. Ibid., pp. 19-20.
32. Ibid., pp. 18-19.
33. Ibid.
34. Hentoff, *A Political Life*.
35. Morris, *The Cost of Good Intentions*, p. 138.
36. Ibid., pp. 90-106.
37. Ibid., pp. 171-203.
38. Ibid., p. 222.
39. Ibid.
40. Ibid., pp. 222-231.
41. Ibid., p. 229.
42. Ibid., pp. 236-237.
43. "Mr. Koch and Other City Choices," *New York Times* (October 25, 1981), p. 18E.
44. Haberman, C., "Koch To Boycott Meeting On City To Avoid Critics," *New York Times* (November 18, 1981), p. B1.
45. Ibid.
46. Morris, *The Cost of Good Intentions*, pp. 236-237.

CHAPTER 2

1. I. Weinstein, "Eighty Years of Public Health in New York City," *Bulletin of the New York Academy of Medicine*, 23, 4:221-223, 1947.

2. J. Blake, *Historical Study of the Development of the New York City Department of Health* (New York: Mayor's Committee on Management Survey, 1950).

3. L. Baumgartner, "One Hundred Years of Health: New York City, 1866-1966," *Bulletin of the New York Academy of Medicine*, 45, 6:555-586, 1969.

4. A. Bushel, *Chronology of New York City Department of Health And Its Predecessor Agencies, 1655-1966* (New York: New York City Department of Health, 1966).

5. J. Duffy, *A History of Public Health in New York City, 1866-1966* (New York: Russell Sage Foundation, 1974).

6. Bushel, *Chronology*, p. 1.

7. Ibid.

8. Baumgartner, "One Hundred Years of Health," p. 556.

9. Bushel, *Chronology*, p. 1.

10. Ibid.

11. Blake, *Historical Study*, p. 3.

12. Bushel, *Chronology*, p. 1.

13. Blake, *Historical Study*, p. 5.

14. Ibid.

15. Bushel, *Chronology*, p. 1.

16. Ibid., p. 2.

17. Ibid., p. 3.

18. Ibid., p. 3.

19. Duffy, *A History*, p. xx.

20. Ibid.

21. Ibid., pp. xx-xxi.

22. Blake, *Historical Study*, p. 19.

23. Ibid., p. 20.

24. Duffy, *A History*, p. 23.

25. Blake, *Historical Study*, p. 22-23.

26. Ibid., p. 19.

27. Ibid., p. 29.

28. Duffy, *A History*, p. 48.

29. Ibid.

30. Ibid.
31. Blake, *Historical Study*, p. 30.
32. Ibid.
33. Duffy, *A History*, p. 67.
34. Blake, *Historical Study*, p. 41.
35. Duffy, *A History*, p. 68.
36. Ibid., p. 78.
37. Ibid., p. 80.
38. Ibid., p. 81.
39. Ibid., p. 82.
40. Ibid., p. 238.
41. Ibid., p. 239.
42. Ibid., p. 241.
43. Bushel, *Chronology*, p. 11.
44. Duffy, *A History*, p. 256.
45. Ibid., p. 257.
46. Ibid., p. 260, Blake, *Historical Study*, p. 61.
47. Bushel, *Chronology*, p. 11.
48. Duffy, *A History*, p. 261.
49. H. Kaufman, *The New York City Health Centers* (University: University of Alabama Press, 1959), p. 2.
50. Ibid., p. 3.
51. Ibid., p. 5.
52. A.C. Mustalish, G. Eidsvold, and L.F. Novick, "Decentralization in the New York City Department of Health: Reorganization of a Public Health Agency," *American Journal of Public Health*, 66, 2:1149-1154, 1976.
53. Kaufman, *The New York City Health Centers*, p. 5.
54. *Annual Report, New York City Board of Health, 1914*, New York, 1915, p. 25.
55. Kaufman, *The New York City Health Centers*, p. 6.
56. Duffy, *A History*, pp. 281-306.
57. Ibid., p. 283.
58. S.J. Baker, *Fighting For Life* (New York: Macmillan, 1939), p. 98.
59. Duffy, *A History*, p. 284.
60. Ibid.
61. Ibid., p. 297.
62. Ibid., p. 294.
63. Ibid., p. 297.

64.   Ibid.
65.   Ibid., p. 307.
66.   Ibid., p. 309.
67.   Blake, *Historical Study,* p. 99.
68.   Duffy, *A History,* p. 310.
69.   C-E. A. Winslow, *The New York Times* (November 17, 1927).
70.   C-E. A. Winslow and S. Zimand, *Health Under the "El", The Story of the Bellevue-Yorkville Health Demonstration in Mid-town, New York* (New York and London: Harper and Bros., 1937).
71.   Blake, *Historical Study,* p. 102.
72.   I.V. Hiscock, *District Health Administration* (Lancaster, Pennsylvania: Science Press Printing Co. 1936), pp. 37-49.
73.   Duffy, *A History,* p. 335.

CHAPTER 3

1.   J. Blake, *Historical Study of the Development of the New York City department of Health* (New York: Mayor's Committee on Management Survey, 1950), p. 106.
2.   J. Duffy, *A History of Public Health in New York City, 1866-1966* (New York: Russell Sage Foundation, 1974), p. 338.
3.   Blake, *Historical Study,* p. 107.
4.   Duffy, *A History,* p. 345.
5.   Ibid.
6.   *District Health Development* (New York: New York City Department of Health, 1939), p. 4.
7.   H. Kaufman, *The New York City Health Centers* (University, University of Alabama Press, 1959), p. 11.
8.   *District Health,* p. 4.
9.   C. F. Bolduan, *Illustrious Contributors to Public Health* (Kingsport, Tennessee: Kingsport Press, 1936), p. 1.
10.   I.V. Hiscock *District Health Administration* (Lancaster, Pennsylvania: Science Press Printing Co., 1936).
11.   Kaufman, *The New York City Health Centers,* p. 12.
12.   Ibid.
13.   Ibid.
14.   Duffy, *A History,* p. 357.
15.   *District Health,* p. 5.

16. Duffy, *A History*, p. 369.
17. Ibid., p. 370.
18. Ibid.
19. E. Stebbins, Personal Interview, February 24, 1981.
20. Duffy, *A History*, p. 372.
21. Kaufman, *The New York City Health Centers*, p. 12.
22. Duffy, *A History*, p. 383.
23. Ibid., p. 387.
24. Ibid.
25. Ibid., p. 388.
26. Ibid.
27. Kaufman, *The New York City Health Centers*, p. 14.
28. Ibid.
29. L. Neugeborn, Personal Interview, February 26, 1981.
30. A. Bushel, *Chronology of New York City Department of Health (New York: New York City Department of Health, 1966), p. 42.*
31. Duffy, *A History*, p. 394.
32. Ibid., p. 396.
33. Ibid.
34. Ibid., p. 401.
35. Ibid., p. 402.
36. *Study of the Department of Health, City of New York For the Mayor's Committee on Management Survey* (New York: American Public Health Association— New York City Department of Health, 1952), p. 9.
37. Kaufman, *The New York City Health Centers*, p. 15.
38. Ibid.
39. Duffy, *A History*, p. 415.
40. Ibid.
41. Ibid., p. 419.
42. Ibid., p. 425.
43. Ibid., p. 428.
44. Ibid.
45. Ibid., p. 435.
46. Ibid., p. 438.
47. Ibid., p. 445.
48. W. Shonick, "Mergers of Public Health Departments With Public Hospitals in Urban Areas," *Medical Care*, Supplement, 18, 8:1-50, 1980.
49. A. Bushel, Personal Interview, February 25, 1981.

50. H. Brown, *Familiar Faces, Hidden Lives* (New York: Harcourt, Brace, Jovanovich, 1976), p. 6.

51. A. Bushel, Personal Interview, February 25, 1981.

52. J.E. Smith, *Guide To The Municipal Government of the City of New York* (New York: Meilen Press, 1973), p. 185.

53. E.J. Kramer, *The New York City Health and Hospitals Corporation: Issues, Problems and Prospects* (Chicago: Hospital Research and Educational Trust, 1977), p. 64.

54. M. Wegman, "Health Departments: Then and Now," *American Journal of Public Health*, 67, 10: 913-914, 1977.

55. Brown, *Familiar Faces, Hidden Lives*, p. 15.

56. Ibid., p. 17.

57. I. Leveson, and J.H. Weiss, *Analysis of Urban Health Problems* (New York: Spectrum Publications, 1976), p. 21.

58. C.R. Morris, *The Cost of Good Intentions: New York City and The Liberal Experiment, 1960-1975* (New York: Norton, 1980), p. 163.

59. W.I. Sayre and H. Kaufman, *Governing New York City: Politics In The Metropolis* (New York: Russell Sage Foundation, 1960), p. 212.

60. Morris, *The Cost of Good Intentions*, p. 163.

CHAPTER 4

1.   C.R. Morris, *The Cost of Good Intentions: New York City and The Liberal Experiment 1960-1975* (New York: Norton, 1980), p. 163.

2.   Ibid., p. 164.

3.   L.E. Bellin, The Fall and Rise of the New York City Department of Health, Address Before the Annual Meeting of the Public Health Association of New York City, May 29, 1974, p. 5.

4.   I. Leveson, and J.H. Weiss, *Analysis of Urban Health Problems* (New York: Spectrum Publications, 1976), p. 19.

5.   Ibid., p. 35.

6.   Ibid., p. 19.

7.   Ibid.

8.   Ibid., p. 20.

9.   Ibid.

10. W.S. Sayre and H. Kaufman *Governing New York City: Politics in the Metropolis* (New York: W.W. Norton and Co.), 1965, p. 232.

11. L.E. Bellin, The Deprofessionalization of the Public Health Agency: Notes on the New Mediocrety, 1974, unpublished manuscript, p. 7.

12. Leveson and Weiss, *Analysis*, p. 14.

13. Ibid., p. 12.

14. A.C. Mustalish, G. Edisvold and L.F. Novick, "Decentralization in the New York City Department of Health: Reorganization of a Public Health Agency," *American Journal of Public Health*, 66, 2:1149-1154, 1976.

15. Leveson and Weiss, *Analysis*, p. 24.

16. Ibid.

17. Ibid.

18. Ibid.

19. Ibid., p. 25.

20. Ibid.

21. Bellin, The Fall and Rise, p. 5.

22. Ibid.

23. Ibid., p. 6.

24. Ibid., p. 4.

25. Ibid.

26. Ibid.

27. Mustalish, Eidsvold, and Novick, Decentralization, p. 1151.

28. Ibid.

29. Ibid.

30. *Health Services Administration, The City of New York, Staff Papers, 1971-1973* (New York: Office of Program Analysis, Planning and Budgeting, 1973).

31. J.H. Weiss, Specifying Research Outcomes In Urban Areas, Paper Presented at the Joint Seminar of Health Services, Research and Health Services Developmental Grants Study Sections, Department of Health, Education and Welfare, January 15, 1975, p. 11.

32. Ibid., p. 10.

33. Ibid., p. 9.

34. Mustalish, Edisvold, and Novick, Decentralization, p. 1151.

35. Ibid.

36. Ibid.

37. Ibid.

38. Ibid., p. 1152.

39. Ibid., p. 1151.

40. Ibid., p. 1152.

41. Ibid.

42. Ibid.

43. Ibid.
44. Ibid.
45. Ibid.
46. Ibid.
47. J. Duffy, *A History of Public Health In New York City: 1866-1966* (New York: Russell Sage Foundation, 1974), p. 297.
48. Morris, *The Cost of Good Intentions*, p. 165.
49. Duffy, *A History*, p. 297.
50. Ibid.

CHAPTER 5

1. L.E. Bellin, The Fall and Rise of the New York City Department of Health, Address Before the Annual Meeting of the Public Health Association of New York City, May 29, 1974, p. 6.
2. Ibid.
3. Ibid., p. 12.
4. Z. Nestlebaum, The Fall and the Fall of the NYCDOH, *Health/Pac*, 83, 84, 85: 5-16, 1979.
5. Ibid., p. 14.
6. P.J. Imperato, "Current Problems of Some New York City Health Agencies," *Bulletin of the New York Academy of Medicine*, 55, 5:463-476, 1979.
7. Ibid., p. 466.
8. Ibid.
9. Local Law 25, City Council, City of New York, May 6, 1977.
10. Executive Order No. 95, Designation of the Commissioner of Health to Succeed to the Powers and Responsibilities of the Health Services Administrator, December 2, 1977.
11. P.J. Imperato, "The New York Swine Influenza Immunization Program," *New Trends and Developments in Vaccines*, A. Voller and H. Friedman, eds., MTP, Lancaster, England, 1978, pp. 71-86.
12. J. Gerston, "Twelve Nutritionists Get Layoff Notice," *The New York Times* (January 18, 1975), p. 37.
13. "Anticipated Impact of Budget Cutbacks on City's Agencies and Municipal Services," *The New York Times* (May 30, 1975), p. 9.
14. L. Dembert, "Beame is Losing Middle Managers," *The New York Times* (September 12, 1976), p. 5.

15. C. Haberman, "Who Cured Fiscal Crisis in the City," *The New York Times* (March 7, 1981), pp.25, 27.

16. A. Mayo, "A Sick Joke. The Collapse of the City Health Department," *The Village Voice* (April 28, 1980), p. 13.

17. Executive Order No. 3, Designation of the Deputy Mayor for Finance to Succeed to the Powers and Responsibilities of the Health Services Administrator and the Deputy Mayor for Intergovernmental Relations to Serve on the Board of Directors of the New York City Health and Hospitals Corporation, January 12, 1978.

18. Executive Order No. 8, Vesting in the Special Advisor to the Mayor on Health Services the Powers and Duties Specified in Chapter 1016 of the Laws of 1969, March 8, 1978.

19. Mayo, Collapse, p. 13.

20. Ibid.

21. R. Blumenthal, "Changes in Milk Dating Bring an Inquiry by City," *The New York Times* (December 29, 1979), pp. 23, 26.

22. Mayo, Collapse, pp. 1, 13-16.

23. Ibid.

24. Sulzberger, A.O., "City Health Department Aims To Reverse Decline," *The New York Times* (October 22, 1981), pp.. B1, B11.

25. Ibid.

26. "Chief Will Quit City Health Post Effective In Fall: Ferrer Says Ill Wife Seeks To Return To Puerto Rico," *The New York Times* (April 7, 1981), p. B7.

27. Sulzberger, City Health.

28. Ibid.

29. Ibid.

30. B. Caress, "The Health of The Hospitals Corporation: The Strange Case of Dr. Kauvar and New York's Municipal Hospitals," *Health Pac*, 12, 6:13-18, 1981.

31. Ibid.

32. R. Sullivan, Ex-Head of Federal Disease Center Named City Health Commissioner," *The New York Times* (November 29, 1981), pp. 1, 40.

CHAPTER 6

1. J. Pfiffner, *Public Administration* (New York: The Ronald Press, Co., 1946), p. 81.

2. *New York City Charter And Administrative Code, 1980-1981 Cumulative Sup-*

plement Annotated (Albany, New York: Williams Press, 1980), Volume 1, pp. 49-60, 1980.

3. H.S. Mustard, *Government In Public Health* (New York: Commonwealth Fund, 1945).

4. F.P. Grad, *Public Health Law Manual* (Washington, D.C.: American Public Health Association, 1975).

5. C.A. Miller et al., "A Survey of Local Public Health Departments And Their Directors," *American Journal of Public Health*, 67, 10: 931-939, 1977.

6. E.F. Brooks et al., "Local Public Health Departments and Their Directors In North Carolina And The United States," *North Carolina Medical Journal*, 37, 6: 293-298, 1976.

7. C.A. Miller et al., "Statutory Authorizations For The Work of Local Health Departments," *American Journal of Public Health*, 67, 10: 940-945, 1977.

8. J.W. Mountain, "Administration of Public Medical Service by Health Departments," *American Journal of Public Health*, 30, 2:138-144, 1940.

9. C-E.A. Winslow, "Who Killed Cock Robin?" *American Journal of Public Health*, 34, 6:658-659, 1944.

10. Miller et al., "A Survey."

11. S. Jonas, "Provision of Public Health Services," in *Preventive Medicine And Public Health*, Eleventh Edition, Edited by John M. Last, ed. (New York: Appleton-Century Crofts, 1980), pp. 1614-1633.

12. L.F. Novick, A. Mustalish and G. Eidsvold, "Converting Child Health Stations To Pediatric Treatment Centers." *Medical Care*, 13, 9: 744-752, 1975.

13. *New York City Charter*, p. 52.

14. Ibid., p. 53.

15. P.J. Imperato, L.M. Drusin, J.S. Marr, B. Topff-Olstein and E. Lambertsen, "The New York City Nurse Epidemiology Program," *Bulletin of The New York Academy of Medicine*, 53, 6:569-585, 1977.

16 J. DeZuane, A. Ashendorff and G. Schaible, *Beach And Harbor Water Sampling Program 1976* (New York: New York City Department of Health, 1977).

17. *New York City Charter*, p. 53.

CHAPTER 7

1. A. Bushel, *Chronology of New York City Department of Health And Its Predecessor Agencies, 1655-1966* (New York: New York City Department of Health, 1966), p. 2.

2. J. Duffy, *A History of Public Health In New York City, 1866-1966* (New York: Russell Sage Foundation, 1974), p. 616.
3. Ibid.
4. Ibid., p. 617
5. Ibid., p. 618
6. Ibid.
7. Ibid.
8. Ibid., p. 619.
9. Ibid., p. 620.
10. J. Blake, *Historical Study of the Development of the New York City Department of Health* (New York: Mayor's Committee on Management Survey, 1950), p. 29.
11. Ibid., p. 30.
12. Duffy, *A History*, p. 356.
13. Ibid., p. 357.
14. *New York City Charter And Administrative Code, 1980-1981 Cumulative Supplement Annotated* Vol. 1 (Albany, New York: Williams Press), p. 49.
15. Ibid., p. 50.
16. Ibid.
17. *Metropolitan Board of Health vs. Heister*, 37 New York 661 (1968); *People ex rel. Cox vs. Justices of the Court of Special Sessions*, 7 Hun 214 (Sup. Ct. 1876).
18. *People vs. Blanchard*, 228 New York 145, 42, N.E. 2d 7 (1942), *Matter of Condon vs. Marshall*, 185 Misc. 638, 641-42, 59 N.Y.S. 2d 52, 55 (Sup. Ct. Kings County, 1945); *Quaker Oats Co. vs. City of New York*, and *Hill Packing Co. vs. City of New York*, 295 N.Y. 527, 539, 68 N.E. 2d 593, 598 (1946).
19. Grossman vs. Baumgartner, 17 N.Y. 2d 345, 271 N.Y.S. 2d 195, 218 N.E. 2d 259 (1966); *Metropolitan Association of Private Day Schools vs. Baumgartner*, 41 Misc. 2d 560, 245 N.Y.S. 2d 733 (Sup. Ct. King County 1963).
20. *Ahlers vs. City of New York*, 59 Misc. 2d 634, 300, N.Y.S. 2d 428 (Sup. Ct. N.Y. County, 1969).
21. *Meat Trade vs. McLaughlin*, 37 Appellate Division, 2d 456, 326 N.Y.S. 2d 683 (1st Dept., 1971).
22. Duffy, *A History*, p. 27.
23. L. Baumgartner and F.P. Grade, "A New Health Code For New York City," *American Journal of Public Health*, 49, 10: 1313-1328, 1959.
24. Article 1, Short Title and General Definitions, *New York City Health Code*, New York, City of New York, 1973, p. 11.

25. Duffy, *A History*, p. 418.
26. Ibid.
27. Baumgartner and Grad, "A New Heath Code," p. 1313.
28. *Annual Report of the Board of Health, City of New York, 1959-1960*, New York, 1960, p. 141.
29. *New York City Health Code*, pp. 2-3.
30. *New York City Charter*, p. 54.
31. Baumgartner and Grad, p. 1315.
32. Ibid.
33. Ibid.
34. Ibid.

CHAPTER 8

1. *New York City Charter And Administrative Code, 1980-1981 Cumulative Supplement Annotated*, Vol 1 (Albany, New York: Williams Press), 1981 p. 49.
2. J. Duffy, *A History of Public Health In New York City 1866-1966* (New York: Russell Sage Foundation, 1974), p. 388.
3. W.S. Sayre and H. Kaufman, *Governing The City: Politics In the Metropolis* (New York: W.W. Norton and Co., 1965), pp. 212-245.
4. Duffy, *A History*, p. 388.
5. *New York City Charter*, p. 49.
6. Bellin, L.E. Googooland And New York City—Comparative Physiology of Two Health Departments, unpublished manuscript, May 25, 1977, p. 10.

CHAPTER 9

1. W.S. Sayre and H. Kaufman *Governing The City: Politics In The Metropolis* (New York: W. W. Norton and Co., 1965), pp. 212-245.
2. W. Shonick, "Health Planning," *Preventive Medicine and Public Health*, Eleventh Edition, John Last, ed. (New York: Appleton-Century-Crofts, 1980), pp. 1545-1613.
3. Ibid.
4. Ibid.
5. M. Bergner, et al., "The Sickness Impact Profile: Conceptual Formulation and Methodology for the Development of a Health Status

Measure," *International Journal of Health Services,* 6: 393-416, 1976.

6. D.L. Sackett, "Evaluation of Health Services," *Preventive Medicine and Public Health,* Eleventh Edition, John Last, ed. (New York: Appleton-Century-Crofts, 1980), pp. 1800-1823.

7. L.E. Bellin, Googooland and New York City—Comparative Physiology of Two Health Departments, unpublished manuscript, May 25, 1977, p. 15.

8. Ibid.

9. Ibid.

10. Ibid., p. 17.

11. Ibid.

12. Ibid.

13. Ibid.

14. Ibid., p. 16.

15. Ibid.

16. D. Harris, P.J. Imperato, and B. Oken, "Dog Bites—An Unrecognized Epidemic," *Bulletin of the New York Academy of Medicine,* 50, 9:981-1000, 1974.

17. Prepared Text of Carter's Farewell Address on Major Issues Facing the Nation, *The New York Times* (January 5, 1981), p. B10.

CHAPTER 10

1. C.R. Morris, *The Cost of Good Intentions: New York City and the Liberal Experiment* (New York: W.W. Norton and Co., 1980), p. 127.

2. Ibid., p. 128.

3. Ibid.

4. Ibid.

5. Ibid.

6. L. Neugeborn, Personal Interview, April 14, 1981.

7. L.E. Bellin, Googooland and New York City—Comparative Physiology of Two Health Departments, unpublished manuscript, May 25, 1977, p. 17.

8. Ibid., p. 18.

9. A. Wildavsky, *The Politics of the Budgetary Process* (Boston: Little, Brown and Co., 1964), p. 14.

10. C.R. Morris, *The Cost of Good Intentions: New York City and the Liberal Experiment* (New York: W.W. Norton and Co., 1980), p. 163.

11. A.O. Bornfriend, "Political Parties and Pressure Groups," *Governing the City: Challenges and Options for New York*, R.H. Connery and D. Caraley, eds. (New York: Frederick A. Praeger, 1969), p. 63.
12. Ibid., p. 64.
13. Ibid., p. 65.
14. Ibid.
15. Bellin, Googooland, p. 29.
16. Ibid., p. 28.
17. Ibid., p. 29.
18. Ibid., p. 31.
19. Ibid., p. 30.
20. Ibid., p. 29.

CHAPTER 11

1. L.E. Bellin, Googooland and New York City—Comparative Physiology of Two Health Departments, unpublished manuscript, May 25, 1977, p. 26.
2. Ibid., p. 27.
3. Ibid.
4. Ibid.
5. Ibid.
6. Ibid., p. 22.
7. Ibid., p. 24.
8. Ibid., p. 27.
9. Ibid., p. 28.
10. C.R. Morris, *The Cost of Good Intentions: New York City and the Liberal Experiment* (New York: W.W. Norton and Co., 1980), p. 163.
11. A.O. Bornfriend, "Political Parties and Pressure Groups," *Governing the City: Challenges and Options for New York,* R.H. Connery and D. Caraley, eds. (New York: Frederick A. Praeger, 1969), p. 63.
12. Ibid., p. 64.
13. Ibid., p. 65.
14. Ibid.
15. Bellin, Googooland, p. 29.
16. Ibid., p. 28.
17. Ibid., p. 29.
18. Ibid., p. 31.

19. Ibid., p. 30.
20. Ibid., p. 29.

CHAPTER 12

1. C.R. Morris, *The Cost of Good Intentions: New York City And The Liberal Experiment* (New York: Norton, 1980), p. 233.
2. Ibid.
3. Ibid.
4. H. Wyatt, "City Hospital Board O.K.'s Plan To Cut Deficit," *New York Daily News* (January 13, 1977), p. 47.
5. Ibid.
6. D. Orin, "Hospitals Battle Hits Critical Point," *Long Island Press* (January 13, 1977), p. 1.
7. Ibid.
8. Wyatt, City Hospital Board.
9. Orin, Hospitals Battle.
10. Ibid.
11. R. Sullivan, "Hospitals Board To Be Convened To Seek The Removal of Holloman," *The New York Times* (January 25, 1977), p. 26.
12. R. Sullivan, "Hospitals Corporation Votes 9 to 7 To Remove Holloman As President," *The New York Times* (January 27, 1977), p. 1.
13. H. Raine, "Hospitals Chief Holloman Ousted by 9 to 7 Vote," *New York Daily News* (January 27, 1977), p. 3.
14. M. Kempton, "Hospitals Board Cuts Its Heart Out," *New York Post*, (January 27, 1977), p. 4.
15. "Holloman Ouster As HHC Head Tacitly Approved by Union," *The Chief* (February 4, 1977), p. 16.
16. Ibid.
17. Ibid.
18. Ibid.
19. H. Wyatt, "Agency Told To List More Hospitals For Ax," *New York Daily News* (March 3, 1977), p. 36.
20. "A Fine Choice," *New York Daily News* (February 17, 1977), p.59.
21. "Gifford May Turn Down Job As Health-Hospitals Boss," *Long Island Press* (February 17, 1977), p. 10.
22. P. Slocum, "Cahill Now Czar for State Health," *Long Island Press* (February 18, 1977), p. 8.
23. Ibid.

24. J. Purnick, "Kevin Cahill, New York's Shadow Governor," *New York Magazine* (July 24, 1978), pp. 47-51.

25. J. Klurfeld, "A Rasputin? Cahill: The Doctor Who Would Be King," *Empire State Report* (July, 1976), pp. 214-217.

26. "Needed: A Health Czar," *New York Daily News* (February 17, 1977), p. 59.

27. L. Greenhouse, "Carey Asks Monitor of City Health Care," *The New York Times* (February 18, 1977), p. 1.

28. "Six Titles In Search of Dr. Pooh-Bah," *The New York Times* (March 29, 1977), p. 30.

29. P.J. Imperato, Personal Diary, February 21, 1977.

30. Ibid., March 3, 1977.

31. Ibid., March 10, 1977.

32. "Grow Up Doc," *New York Daily News* (March 12, 1977), p. 19.

33. Ibid.

34. L.E. Bellin, "The Health Czar And The Long, Long Chain," *New York Daily News* March 15, 1977), p. 30.

35. Ibid.

36. "Dr. Cahill Named to Board of Health," *The New York Times* (June 13, 1981), p. 27.

37. R. Sullivan, "Board Authority Set For New Health Post By Beame And Carey: Job Combining Six Positions Would Oversee Hospitals In The City To Rationalize The System," *The New York Times* (March 28, 1977), p. 1.

38. P. Meskil and H. Wyatt, "Health Czar Is Rx For City," *New York Daily News* (March 28, 1977), p. 13.

39. "City Health Boss Balks At Plan To Give Him Boss," *Staten Island Advance* (March 28, 1977), p. 2.

40. Six Titles.

41. "The New Health Czar," *New York Daily News* (March 29, 1977), p. 33.

42. P. Kihss, "Carey-Beame Proposal To Create City Health Chief Is 'Condemned'," *The New York Times* (April 17, 1977), p. 47.

43. Ibid.

44. H.C. McCall, "To Your Health," *Amsterdam News* (March 5, 1977), p. 16.

45. D. Yuncker, "Health Czar Plan: Complications Develop," *New York Post* (April 15, 1977), p. 24A.

46. R. Sullivan, "Beame Is Expected To Move Today To Tighten Rule Over Hospital Unit," *The New York Times* (April 26, 1977), p. 1.

47. B. Yuncker, "Vote Due On Plan For Hospital Reins," *New York Post* (April 26, 1977), p. 2.

48. R. Sullivan, "Hospitals' New Regimen: Ousters And Shifts Under Two Leaders Named By Beame May Ease Way To A State Health Czar," *The New York Times* (April 30, 1977), p. 35.

49. R. Sullivan, "Beame's Fiscal Aide Gets Hospital Post: Kummerfeld Will Head Committee That Will Run The System—Takeover By Mayor Seen," *The New York Times* (April 27, 1977), p. 32.

50. Yuncker, Vote Due.

51. R. Sullivan, "Carey Expected To Announce Today A Post For Containing Health Costs," *The New York Times* (May 3, 1977), p. 37.

52. H. Wyatt, "City Health Czar Candidates Down To 4 But Job's In Peril," *New York Daily News* (May 12, 1977), p. 18.

53. R. Sullivan, "Health Chief Sought By Beame And Carey: But Mayor And Governor Are Unable To Agree On Choice To Supervise Consolidation of Hospitals," *The New York Times* (June 6, 1977), p. 33.

54. Ibid.

55. Ibid.

56. R. Sullivan, "Carey Choice For A 'Health Czar' Is Resisted By Beame And Koch," *The New York Times* (September 24, 1977), p. 24.

57. R. Sullivan, " 'Health Czar' Appointed By Carey Finds City A 'Shoestring' Empire," *The New York Times* (November 7, 1977), p. 39.

58. H. Wyatt, "Carey Chooses Medicaid Expert As 1st Health Car," *New York Daily News* (September 23, 1977), p. 3.

59. R. Sullivan, "Cahill Quits Job As Medical Aide On Carey's Staff," *The New York Times* (December 16, 1980), p. B5.

60. B. Yuncker and A. Greenspan, "Two of Gov. Carey's Top Personal Aides Throw In The Towel," *New York Post* (December 16, 1980), p. 7.

CHAPTER 13

1. A.P. Sanoff, "Uneasy Press Sets Out to Refurbish Its Image," *U..S. and World Report*, XC, 25: 71-72, 1981.

2. Ibid.

3. Ibid.

4. Ibid.

5. Ibid.

6. Ibid.

7. Ibid.

8. S. Molotsky, "Carter Decides Against Suing for Libel," *The New York Times* (October 25, 1981), p. 26.

9. P. Gauley, "Carter May Drop Plans To Sue Paper for Libel," *The New York Times* (October 24, 1981), p. 10.

10. Ibid.

11. Molotsky, op. cit.

12. Ibid.

13. Text of Statement On Paper's Apology, *The New York Times* (October 25, 1981), p. 27

14. Ibid.

15. Ibid.

16. Ibid.

17. J. Friendly, "Notebook: 3 Criticisms For Editors," *The New York Times* (October 25, 1981), p. 31.

18. Sanoff, op. cit.

19. Ibid.

20. Ibid.

ABOUT THE AUTHOR

Pascal James Imperato, M.D. is a specialist in preventive medicine and public health. After receiving his M.D. degree from the State University of New York, Downstate Medical Center in 1962, he completed his internship and residency in internal medicine at the Long Island College Hospital in New York City. In 1966 he received an M.P.H. & T.M. degree from Tulane University's School of Public Health and Tropical Medicine. From 1966 to 1972 he was a medical epidemiologist with the Center for Disease Control of the U.S. Public Health Service, assigned to the West African country of Mali. Beginning in 1972 he successively served in the New York City Department of Health as Director of the Bureau of Infectious Disease Control and First Deputy Commissioner, being appointed Commissioner of Health, and Acting Health Services Administrator in 1977. From 1977 to 1978 he also served as Chairman of the Board of Directors of the New York City Health and Hospitals Corporation. Since 1978, Dr. Imperato has been Professor and Chairman of the Department of Preventive Medicine and Community Health, State University of New York, Downstate Medical Center and Adjunct Profesor of Public Health at The Cornell University Medical College.

INDEX